Musculoskeletal Disorders at Work

Musculoskeletal Disorders at Work

Proceedings of a conference held at
The University of Surrey, Guildford
13–15 April 1987

Edited by
Peter Buckle
The Robens Institute, Guildford

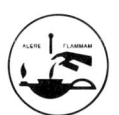

Taylor & Francis
London • New York • Philadelphia
1987

UK	Taylor & Francis Ltd, 4 John St, London WC1N 2ET
USA	Taylor & Francis Inc, 242 Cherry St, Philadelphia, PA 19106-1906

Copyright © Taylor & Francis Ltd 1987

All rights reserved. No part of this publication may be reproduced, stored in a retrieval system, or transmitted in any form or by any means, electronic, mechanical, photocopying, recording or otherwise, without permission in writing from the publisher.

British Library Cataloguing in Publication Data
Musculoskeletal disorders at work :
  proceedings of a conference held at the
  University of Surrey, Guildford, 13-15
  April 1987.
  1. Musculoskeletal system——Wounds and
  injuries 2. Industrial accidents
  I. Buckle, Peter
  617'.47044   RD732

ISBN 0-85066-381-4

Printed in Great Britain by Taylor & Francis (Printers) Ltd, Basingstoke, Hants.

CONTENTS

Introduction   7

A Review of Epidemiological Research on Risk
Factors of Low Back Pain
Hildebrandt, V.   9

Physical Work Environment and Musculoskeletal
Disorders in the Busdriver's Profession
*Kompier, M., de Vries, M., van Noord, F.,
Mulders, H., Meijman, T. and Broersen, J.*   17

Physical Work Load and Musculoskeletal Disorders
in the Engineering Industry
Leino, P. and Hasan, J.   23

The Spinal Engine and Its Gearbox
Gracovetsky, S. and Carbone, A.   25

Computer-Aided Analysis of Trunk and Shoulder Posture
Keyserling, W.M., Fine, L.J. and Punnett, L.   31

Arm-lift Strength Variation Due to Task Parameters
Kumar, S.   37

Portable Microcomputer Based Technique for Posture
or Activity Recording in the Field
Clark, A.G., Browne, K., Madeley, R. and Ridd, J.E.   43

Evaluation of Work Posture.1. A Model for
Evaluation of Seated Work Tasks
Eklund, J.A.E., Zettergren, S. and Odenrick, P.   50

Contents

Evaluation of Work Postures. 2. Measurement and Analysis of Work Postures in the Field
Odenrick, P., Eklund, J.A.E., Zettergren, S. and Örtengren, R. ... 56

Evaluation of Work Postures. 3. Workplace Design for Crane Drivers in a Steelworks
Zettergren, S., Eklund, J.A.E. and Odenrick, P. ... 62

One Year's Notifications of Back Injuries to the National Society Security Office, Especially with Respect to Nature of Cause, Medical Diagnoses and Consequences
Josefsen, K., Boss, A.H., Andersen, V. and Biering-Sorensen, F. ... 68

An Epidemiologic Study of Postural Risk Factors for Back Disorders in Industry
Punnett, L., Fine, L.J. and Keyerling, W.M. ... 74

Risk factors in Back Pain
Porter, R.W. ... 75

One Year's Notifications of Back Injuries to the National Social Security Office. A Demographic Description
Andersen, V., Boss, A.H., Josefsen, K. and Biering-Sorensen, F. ... 82

Working Postures and Spinal Diseases among Porphyry Quarrymen
Colombini, D., Occhipinti, E., Cristofolini, A. and Grieco, A. ... 89

Shovel Design and Back Load in Digging Trenches
van der Grinten, M. ... 96

Stature Changes and Psychophysical Ratings Associated with Repetitive Lifting
Vincent, M., Buckle, P.W. and Stubbs, D.A. ... 102

An Epidemiological Study of Postural Risk Factors for Shoulder Disorders in Industry
Fine, L.J., Punnett, L. and Keyserling, W.M. ... 108

Contents

Neck and Shoulder Complaints Among Sewing-machine Operators. Frequencies and Diagnoses in Comparison to a Control Population
Bläder, S., Barch Holst, U., Danielsson, S., Ferhm, F., Kalpamaa, M., Leijon, K., Lindh, M., Markhede, G. and Mikaelsson, B. 110

RSI - The Australian Experience
Meyer, R.H. 112

A Review of Research on Repetitive Strain Injuries (RSI)
Bammer, G. and Blignault, I. 118

Carpal Tunnel Syndrome and Associated Risk Factors - A Review
Turner, J.P. and Buckle, P.W. 124

Conservative Management of Carpal Tunnel Syndrome Utilizing Pyridoxine
Kasdan, M.L. 133

A National Strategy for the Prevention and Management of RSI
Liddicoat, K. and Ellis, N. 139

Prevention of Injuries Related to Physical Stress through Intervention by Labour Inspectors
Kemmlert, K., Kilbom, Å., Nilsson, B., Andersson, R. and Bjurvald, M. 146

Repetitive Strain Injuries among Service Personnel on North Sea Oil Platforms
Waersted, M. and Westgaard, R.H. 153

Training in Safe Lifting: Are the Methods Taught Used by Workers?
St-Vincent, M., Lortie, M. and Tellier, C. 159

Tests of Manual Working Capacity and the Prediction of Low Back Pain
Troup, J.D.G., Foreman, T.K., Baxter, C.E. and Brown, D. 165

Three Dimensional Non-Invasive Assessment of Lumbar Brace Immobilization of the Spine
Dorsky, S., Buchalter, D., Kahanovitz, N. and Nordin, M. 171

The Use of the Hettinger Test in Pre-employment Screening
Thompson, D., Lowerson, A. and Zalewski, M. 177

Reducing Upper Limb Strain Injury by Redesign: A Case Study in the Food Processing Industry
Mabey, M.H., Pethick, A.J., Graves, R.J. and Adams, P.K. 183

Reducing Repetitive Strain and Back Pain among Bricklayers
Akinmayowa, N.K. 189

Musculoskeletal Disorders among Cargo Handlers
Akinmayowa, N.K. and Akintunji, I. 194

An International Comparison of the Prevalence of RSI among Keyboard Operators and its Relationship to Office Work Practices
Bammer, G. 200

Integrated Biomechanical Examination of the Musculoskeletal System
Byfield, D. 201

Comparative Analysis of Electrical Stimulation and Exercises to Increase Trunk Muscle Strength and Endurance
Kahanovitz, N., Nordin, M., Viola, K., Yabut, S., Parnianpour, M. and Mulvihill, M. 213

The Low-back Pain Prevailing among the Freight-container Tractor Drivers in Japan
Nakata, M., Nishiyama, K. and Watanabe, S. 221

Introduction of Standing Aids in the Furniture Industry
Nijboer, I. and Dul, J. 227

Correlation between Different Tests of Trunk Strength
Parnianpour, M., Nordin, M., Moritz, U. and Kahanovitz, N. 234

Development of a Practical Method for Workplace Redesign to Reduce Upper Limb Strain Injury
Pethick, A.J., Mabey, M.H. and Graves, R.J. 239

Contents

Patient Lifting: An Ergonomic Approach
Poll, K.J. 247

Musculoskeletal Problems in Supermarket Workers
Ryan, G.A. 250

Postural Factors, Work Organization, and Musculo-skeletal Symptoms
Ryan, G.A., Hage, B. and Bampton, M. 251

Musculoskeletal Disorders at Work in Building Construction: Epicondylitis and Low Back Pain
Salengro, B. and Commandre, F. 254

Author Index 259

Subject Index 261

INTRODUCTION

The following collection of papers formed the basis of the conference entitled 'Musculoskeletal Disorders at Work' held at the University of Surrey in April 1987. The conference was organised in the hope of bringing together an international group of researchers to consider the nature of these disorders which are so costly and cause such suffering to so many groups of workers around the world.

In the event, more than 40 scientific papers were selected from researchers representing five continents, thereby providing a global state of the art profile.

The order of the presentation of papers has been planned to consider the following aspects:- the epidemiology of general musculoskeletal disorders, the methods for assessment of both exposure and outcome variables, studies of particular disorders (e.g. back pain, RSI, shoulder disorders, carpal tunnel syndrome) and a consideration of possible preventative strategies including training, selection, screening and ergonomic design. A number of papers also consider other aspects of management of the problem and old and new methods of treatment are examined.

Specific occupations which have been investigated include:- bus drivers, crane operators, quarrymen, sewing machinists, clerical workers, keyboard operators, hospital staff, oil rig personnel, construction workers, cargo handlers and freight container tractor drivers. The resultant international mix of static and dynamic, manual and sedentary, high stress and low stress, male and female employment ensures that the proceedings are both stimulating and challenging for researchers and practitioners alike.

In compiling these proceedings it has become apparent to me that despite, or perhaps because of, the wide range of backgrounds, resources and disciplines of the contributors, common approaches and answers are being found. I hope that this conference will further these shared goals.

Peter Buckle, April 1987.

A REVIEW OF EPIDEMIOLOGICAL RESEARCH ON RISK FACTORS OF LOW BACK PAIN

Vincent H. HILDEBRANDT

TNO Institute of Preventive Health Care,
P.O.Box 124
NL-2300 AC Leiden, The Netherlands

ABSTRACT
   A review of epidemiological studies on risk factors of low back pain was carried out, using five recent comprehensive publications on low back pain. Fifty-four individual risk factors were mentioned, often only by one or two sources. References were often small. In general, the sources consulted agreed with respect to the following six individual risk factors: age, relative muscle strength, physical fitness, back complaints in the past, psychosocial factors in general and work experience. Twenty-three work-related factors were mentioned, including general factors (e.g. heavy physical work and manual handling), static working postures (e.g. sitting), dynamic workload (e.g. lifting), pushing/ pulling, trunk rotation, and environmental factors (e.g. vibrations). Again, the number of references was small.
It is concluded that the interpretation of the vast amount of epidemiological data on the correlates of low back pain is still difficult and confusing. Possible explanations are discussed with special attention to methodological problems which should be solved in future epidemiologic research.

INTRODUCTION
   Over the past 30 years, numerous epidemiological studies on work-related musculoskeletal disorders have been published, especially on the low back. Life-time prevalence of low back problems is known to be high, exceeding 50% in the general population (Valkenburg & Haanen 1982). In certain occupations almost nine out of ten workers do experience low back pain once in their lives (e.g. Riihimäki 1985). Thus it is not surprising that the need for effective preventive actions is stressed over and over

again. Epidemiology is one of the contributors of knowledge necessary to develop such actions. In particular the identification of individual and work-related risk factors can be relevant for the prevention of musculoskeletal disease, providing basic information for taking specific preventive actions. To obtain a summary of risk factors identified until now, a review study was performed and results were evaluated especially from a methodological point of view.

METHOD

To avoid analyzing thousands of articles, five recent comprehensive publications on low back pain were analysed. The five sources consisted of three books (Jayson 1980, White & Gordon 1982, Pope et al 1984) and two review-articles (Yu 1984, Troup 1984). These sources were selected from a long list of recent publications on the low back because they gave an up-to-date summary and interpretation of epidemiologic studies on low back pain by well-known international experts. Together these five sources were considered to give a valid picture of the "state of the art". Previously, a part of this review was used in a study on ergonomic guidelines for the prevention of low back pain at the workplace, reported elsewhere (Dul & Hildebrandt 1987). Potential risk factors mentioned in the sources were identified and it was determined whether a factor was considered within the source to be associated with low back pain or not. Also, the number of references given by the source was analysed. Comparison of the results of the five sources together resulted in a comprehensive list of mentioned risk factors.

In a follow-up study, a detailed analysis of all basic studies will be performed.

RESULTS

Table 1 shows individual risk factors mentioned in one or more of the five sources, categorised into constitutional, postural-structural, radiographic, medical, psychosocial, demographic and other factors (after Frymoyer, 1984).

Table 1. Possible individual risk factors of low back pain, mentioned in at least one of five epidemiological sources.

---

constitutional
age, sex, height, weight, back muscle strength (absolute and relative), fitness, back mobility, genetic factors
postural-structural
severe scoliosis, difference in length of legs
radiographic
severe multi-level degeneration, disc resorption, disc herniation, severe arthrosis facets, spondylarthropathies, spondylolysis, spondylolisthesis, sacralisation/transitional vertebra, skeletal defects, fractures, neoplasmata, severe kyphosis, lumbar kyphosis, infectious diseases, gravities
medical
back complaints in the past, number of births and gravities
psychosocial
depression, anxiety, 'life events', family problems, divorce, personality, hypochondriasis, somatization, disssatisfaction with work or social status of work, tense and fatigued after work, high degree of responsibility and mental concentration, poorer intellectual capacity, lesser ability to establish emotional contacts, lesser 'philosophic' attitude
demographic
social-economic situation, educational level, location of home
other
sports, degree of physical activity, gardening, caring for grandchildren, smoking, alcohol, coughing, workexperience

---

Fifty-five individual risk factors were identified. Besides these, an additional eightteen factors were mentioned which were regarded as non-risk factors. These factors included body build, height/weight indexes, etnical factors, kyphosis, lordosis, aspecific radiographic abnormalities, radiographic findings like Schmorl's nodes, osteophytes, disc narrowing, facet-asymmetry, spina bifida occulta, osteoporosis, lordosis, scoliosis and increased lumbo-sacral angle, severe mental problems like psychosis and neurosis as well as marital status.

Most factors (74%) were only mentioned in one or two sources and references were often small. Therefore factors were selected which were mentioned by at least three sources and might thus be considered as 'generally accepted' risk factors of low back pain (Table 2).

Table 2. Risk factors of low back pain mentioned in at least three of five epidemiological sources.

constitutional	age
	relative muscle strength
	physical fitness
medical	back complaints in the past
psychosocial factors	not specified
others	work experience

Age, relative muscle strength (the ratio between job requirements and individual capacity), physical fitness, back complaints in the past, psychosocial factors in general and work experience appeared to be generally accepted risk factors. Aspecific radiographic abnormalities were considered of no importance by almost all sources.

Hence, of a total of seventy-three individual factors mentioned, only six individual characteristics were rather consistently described as risk-factors and one as non-risk factor.

Table 3 shows the work-related risk factors, categorised into static and dynamic work, factors in the working environment and factors concerning the content of the work.

Table 3. Possible work-related risk factors for low back pain mentioned in at least one of five different epidemiological sources.

general
heavy physical work, working postures in general
static work load
static working postures in general, prolonged sitting, standing or stooping, reaching, no variation of working posture
dynamic work load
heavy manual handling, lifting (heavy or frequent, unexpected heavy, infrequent, torque), carrying, forward flexion of trunk, rotation of trunk, pushing/ pulling
working environment
vibrations, jolts, slipping/falling
work content
monotony, repetitive work, work dissatisfaction

Twenty-four work-related factors were found which were regarded as risk factors by one or more sources. Only one factor (climate) was said to be no risk factor (by one source). Factors mentioned by at least three sources are shown in table 4.

Table 4. Work-related risk factors of low back pain, mentioned by at least three of five epidemiological sources.

---

general
heavy physical work
static work load
prolonged sitting
dynamic work load
heavy manual handling, heavy or frequent lifting, trunk rotating, pushing/pulling
work environment
vibrations

Heavy work in general, prolonged sitting, heavy manual handling, heavy or frequent lifting, rotating, pushing/pulling and vibrations are work related risk factors which could be regarded as 'generally accepted'. Considering the work-related factors, more agreement could be noted between the sources, although again the number of references was often small.

Of all ninety-eight factors involved (both individual and work-related), 22% had no reference and 48% had only one reference.

DISCUSSION

The review resulted in a list of seventy-three individual factors and twenty-five work-related factors which have been considered as potential risk factors of low back pain. Most factors were mentioned only in one or two sources (74%). Assuming that a certain degree of agreement between the sources is an indication of the importance of the factor involved, it was analysed which factors were considered risk factors in at least three of the five sources. Only six individual factors (11%) and eight work-related factors (33%) did survive such a restriction (see tables 2 and 4). Hence, it appears that the interpretation of the results of epidemiological studies is difficult and confusing, apparently leading to different conclusions.

A number of methodological difficulties can at least partially explain this interpretation-problem. They involve the study-designs, study-populations, measures of exposure and -effect, the number and nature of risk factors considered and the method of analysis used.

A great variety of populations is used for epidemiological studies. Data-sources on large populations are often incomplete and (occupational) subgroups ill-defined. Clinical and occupational populations constitute even greater selections, since clinical populations contain more 'serious' cases and occupational populations less 'serious' cases. Data which have been gathered for insurance reasons (most sick-leave- and accident data) can be severely biased when musculoskeletal problems are considered a legal reason for claims (e.g. Klein 1984).

Most studies are cross-sectional, not permitting differentiation between cause and effect or evaluation of the predictive value of correlates of musculoskeletal disorders.

It is not yet clear which exposure-variables are relevant. This has resulted in a great variety of measures, often restricted to global descriptions at the level of industrial sector or occupation. Such measures do not give sufficient insight in relevant tasks or working conditions. Quantification of working aspects is rarely performed. Often, no data are available on duration of exposure in the present and past job(s). The exposition to combinations of different types of workloads is seldomly assessed.

Since a valid and international accepted classification system for low back pain is not available, effect-measures show a great variety too, ranging from detailed clinical diagnosis to simple registration of complaints (Buckle 1985, Anderson 1986). Reproducable quantified measures are still lacking.

The nature and amount of risk factors considered in the different studies varies considerably. The same is true for the way in which these factors are quantified. It appears that many potential risk factors simply are not studied specifically enough to allow valid conclusions. Climate is an example: it is generally considered as a risk factor of musculoskeletal problems, but not identified as such in the literature. Other factors are studied more specifically, but in only a few studies, which askes for some reserve in interpretation. Examples of such factors are the relative muscle strength and physical fitness as individual risk factors for low back pain.

Many studies, particularly older studies, present crude results, without corrections for potential confounders or interaction between variables, which makes interpretation of the results almost impossible.

The main consequence of these methodological problems is a lack of comparability of studies which prevents obtaining a valid overall picture of the various findings. This has resulted in an uncertainty about relevant risk factors and their predictive value. Future research has to deal with those methodological problems in order to facilitate interpretation and usefulness of study-results. Attention has to be paid in particular to controlled and prospective studies, representativeness of study-populations, definition and quantification of exposure- and effect-variables, enabling identification of dose-effect relationships as well as multivariate analysis including potential interactive or confounding factors.

Reviewing recent studies, several promising trends can be observed. Standardization of questionnaires on musculo-skeletal complaints (Johnnson 1984), attempts to quantify physical effects variables (e.g. Smith 1985) and exposure variables (e.g. Kilbom 1986) as well as longitudinal studies (e.g. Biering-Sörensen 1983) are gradually adding new and relevant knowledge. Reinforcement of this kind of epidemiologic research seems important as materials for a comprehensive preventive approach for work-related musculo-skeletal morbidity.

CONCLUSION

Epidemiological research has identified many potential individual and work related risk factors of low back pain. However, interpretation appears to be difficult and confusing. Particularly some methodological problems hamper comparability between studies and validity of the results. Furthermore, to allow definitive conclusions on the significance of a individual or work-related characteristic as a risk factor of low back pain, many factors do not seem to be studied specifically enough. Nevertheless, the following factors appear to be most important: age, relative muscle strength, physical fitness, back complaints in the past, psychosocial problems in general and work-experience as individual risk factors and heavy physical work, heavy manual handling, prolonged sitting postures, heavy or frequent lifting, rotating of the trunk, pushing/pulling and vibrations as work-related risk factors.

ACKNOWLEDGEMENT

This study has been initiated and financially supported by the Dutch Ministry of Social Affairs and Employment.

REFERENCES

Anderson, J.A.D. 1986 Epidemiological aspects of back pain *Journal of the Society of Occupational Medicine* 36, 90-94.

Biering-Sørensen, F 1983 A prospective study of low back pain in a general population *Scandinavian Journal of Rhabilitation Medicine* 15, 71-79.

Buckle, P.W. et al 1985 Identification of risk factors associated with musculo-skeletal disorders. In *Ergonomics International 85*; proceedings of the ninth Congress of the International Ergonomics Association, 2-6 September 1985, Bournemouth, England, edited by I.D.Brown et al (Taylor & Francis London).

Dul, J & Hildebrandt, V.H. 1987 Ergonomic guidelines for the prevention of low back pain at the workplace, *Ergonomics* (in press).

Frymoyer, J.W. 1984 Helping your patient avoid low back pain *Journal of Musculoskeletal Medicine* 1, 65-74.

Jayson, M.I.V.(ed) 1980, *The lumbar spine and back pain*. 2nd edition. (Pitman).

Kilbom, A et al 1986 Disorders of the cervicobrachial regio among female workers in the electronics industry *International Journal of Industrial Ergonomics* 1, 37-47.

Klein, B.P. et al 1984 Assessment of workers' compensation claims for back strains/sprains *Journal of Occupational Medicine* 26, 443-448.

Pope, M.H. et al (eds), 1984 *Occupational Low Back Pain*, (Praeger).

Riihimäki, H 1985 Backpain and heavy physical work: a comparative study of concrete reinforcement workers and maintenance house painters *British Journal of Industrial Medicine* 42, 226-232.

Smith, S.S. et al 1985 Quantification of lumbar function part I: Isometric and mutispeed isokinetic trunk strength measures in sagittal and axial planes in normal subjects *Spine* 10, 757-772.

Troup, J.D.G., 1984 Causes, prediction and prevention of back pain at work. *Scandinavian Journal of Work Environment & Work* 10, 419-428.

Valkenburg, H.A. & Haanen, H.L.M. 1982 The epidemiology of low back pain In: *Symposium on idiopathic low back pain* edited by A.A. White & S.L. Gordon (The C.V. Mosby Company).

White, A.A.W. & Gordon, S.L. (eds) 1982 *Symposium in idiopathic low back pain* (The C.V.Mosby Company)

Yu, T. et al, 1984 Low back pain in industry - an old problem revisited *Journal of Occupational Medicine* 517-524.

PHYSICAL WORK ENVIRONMENT AND MUSCULOSKELETAL
DISORDERS IN THE BUSDRIVER'S PROFESSION

M. Kompier, M. de Vries, F. van Noord,
H. Mulders, T. Meijman, J. Broersen

Institute for Experimental & Occupational Psychology
University of Groningen, The Netherlands

ABSTRACT

Both medical disablement figures and the amount of musculoskeletal complaints indicate that musculoskeletal disorders are a major work-related health problem in Dutch city-busdrivers.
It is hypothesised that poor ergonomics of the city buscabin and inconveniences in the physical work environment and work strain are systematically related to (self-reported) musculoskeletal disorders.

INTRODUCTION

Dutch city busdrivers show relatively high absenteeism figures and a disablement expectation that is twice as high as the average of other Dutch male civil servants (Kompier et al., 1986). According to medical insurance authorities, main reasons for medical unfitness are musculoskeletal disorders (35% of all medically disabled drivers versus 19.5% of all male civil servants; period 1977-1984). Among city busdrivers disorders of the back, the neck, the tendons and joints and of connective tissue are the most prominent ones in this category.
It was decided to study the ergonomics of the standard city buscabin (ergonomic study, ergonomic survey) and self-reported musculoskeletal disorders of city busdrivers in Groningen, a Dutch provincial capital with 168.000 inhabitants.

ERGONOMICS OF THE STANDARD CITY BUSCABIN[1]

A representative sample - stratified towards year of construction - of 14 standard city buses (DAF company, chassis type SB-201, coachwork Hainje Heerenveen) of the municipal bus company is studied.

It is demonstrated that there is no uniformity in the design and construction of various cabin components.

Moreover, several shortcomings are reported, in particular concerning driving seat (no adjustable springs, no adjustable lumbar support, insufficient vertical adjustability), steering wheel (fixed, diameter too large, angle of inclination - 12°- too limited), pedals and working area.

It is demonstrated that, as a result of these deficiencies, drivers are not able to obtain an adequate adjustment of seat, steering wheel and pedals, fitting individual anthropometric characteristics.

ERGONOMIC SURVEY: PHYSICAL WORK ENVIRONMENT AND WORK STRAIN

In order to further identify occupational hazards in the busdriver's profession two questionnaires are administered among all city busdrivers in Groningen (response 73%; 158 male, 10 female; mean age 33.7 (sd.8.0) mean years of service 7.7 (sd.6.2).

Both the physical work environment scale, 17 items, and the work strain scale, 15 items, are highly reliable scales (Dijkstra et al., 1981).

Reference groups are 655 busdrivers (city of Rotterdam, Oversloot et al., 1982), 315 white collar workers and 1800 blue collar workers, all in executive service (Dijkstra et al., 1981). Busdrivers in both cities are of comparable age. Reference groups are older (Table 1).

Table 1. Age distribution busdrivers in Groningen and reference groups.

	n	17-34	35-49	50-65
City busdrivers Groningen	168*	56%	39%	5%
City busdrivers Rotterdam	992**	50%	39%	11%
White collar workers	407***	33%	39%	28%
Blue collar workers	2036	39%	33%	28%

* including 235 tram drivers and 102 subway drivers.
** including 92 staff members.
*** including 236 staff members.

Table 2. Working environment and work strain.
Proportions of workers with complaints;
only items with proportions > 30% are shown.
χ^2-test testing differences with busdrivers
Groningen (df:1) *p<0.05, **p<0.01, ***p<0.001.

	City bus Groningen n=168	City bus R'dam n=655[1]	White collar n=315[2]	Blue collar n=1800[2]
Phys.working environm.				
Lot of inconvenience by				
- draft, wind	85%	87%	20%***,**	45%**,***
- change of temperature	80%	86%	21%***	51%***
- vibration	74%	81%**	4%***	15%***
- dry air	64%	51%	32%***	26%***
- cold	52%	49%	17%***	23%
- noise	52%	47%	16%***	53%***
- bad smell	52%	47%	7%***	37%***
- heat	46%	39%	21%	23%
- bad illumination, blinding, reflection	44%	46%**	10%***	14%***
- dust	44%	11%	7%***	37%***
- vapour, mist, gas	40%	43%	3%	27%***
- lack of fresh air	31%	31%	32%***	47%***
- wet air, rain	27%	34%**	8%***	12%
- dirt, grease	25%	15%	3%	32%
- bad layout workstation	43%	52%*	12%***	38%
Work strain				
- should actually slow down	50%	34%***	21%***	26%***
- trouble with intently looking at	38%	13%***	11%***	17%***
- labour often too tiring	34%	25%*	31%***	37%***
- trouble with sitting	34%	24%	7%	6%
- trouble with working in uncomfortable body posture	17%	13%	6%***	32%***

1. Oversloot et al., 1982.
2. Dijkstra et al., 1981.

On particular items a strong agreement is shown between city busdrivers in two different cities. Furthermore large differences are demonstrated between these drivers and administrative and industrial reference groups. Therefore, four major occupational hazards can be demonstrated:
- vibration
- climatological factors
- bad illumination, blinding, reflection
- forced seating position during work (static work load); trouble with sitting is a common complaint for both groups of drivers, even though it is more common among busdrivers in Groningen.

SELF REPORTED MUSCULOSKELETAL DISORDERS

The same 168 drivers answered a questionnaire on musculoskeletal complaints (Andersson & Ydreborg, 1984; Cronbach's α in our study 0.75).

Table 3 shows the answers of 158 male city busdrivers and of a reference group of 2728 male Swedish workers - whose age distribution unfortunately is not known - in various occupations.

Table 3. Self reported musculoskeletal disorders and absence frequency (at least once during the last year) due to these disorders in percentages. City busdrivers and a reference group.
χ^2-test (with df:1) *p<0.05, **p<0.01, ***p<0.001.

	Reported disorders Bus(n=158)	Ref.group[1] (n=2728)	Rep.abs.freq. Bus	Ref.gr.
Lower part of back	57%***	40%	20%*	14%
Neck	44%***	23%	18%***	4%
Shoulders	42%***	21%	13%	5%
Upper part of back	28%***	9%	11%***	3%
Knees	27%	23%	5%	5%
Upper arms	23%	-[2]	7%	-[2]
Ankles and knees	20%*	13%	4%	4%
Hips and thighs	15%	10%	7%*	3%
Calfs	14%	-[2]	1%	-[2]
Wrists and hands	9%	10%	3%	2%
Elbows	8%	9%	3%	2%

1. Andersson & Ydreborg, 1984.
2. No data available.

During the last 12 months musculoskeletal disorders have been reported by 82% of all drivers; 48% of these men (40% of all drivers) also report having been absent from work at least once due to these disorders.

The four most frequently reported disorders - lower part of back, neck, shoulders, upper part of back - are mentioned significantly more among busdrivers.

The incidence of self reported absence frequency due to these disorders is also higher among busdrivers.

Self reported musculoskeletal disorders (sumscore) are systematically related to the physical work environment scores (pearson r 0.41) and to the work strain score (pearson r 0.49).

The relationship between age and amount of self reported musculoskeletal disorders, as well as that between years of

service as a busdriver and these complaints is shown in
Figure 1. Age and years of service are intercorrelated .86
(pearson r).

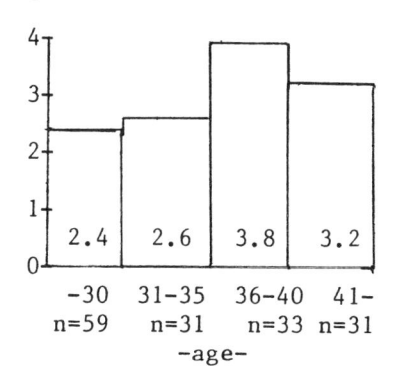

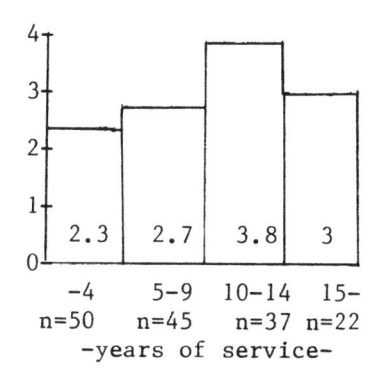

```
 4                                      4
 3                                      3
 2                                      2
 1  2.4  2.6  3.8  3.2                  1  2.3  2.7  3.8   3
 0                                      0
   -30  31-35 36-40 41-                   -4   5-9  10-14 15-
   n=59 n=31  n=33  n=31                  n=50 n=45 n=37  n=22
           -age-                              -years of service-
```

Figure 1. Relationships between age and years of service
and self reported musculoskeletal disorders
amongst male busdrivers.

Disorders are reported increasingly more frequently
until the fourth time period. In the oldest time periods the
amount of complaints decreases. Still it is stays higher
compared with the two youngest time periods.
Statistically, both age and years of service show a
significant influence on musculoskeletal complaints
($F(3,150)$= 3.2; p= 0.025 and ($F(3,150)$= 3.64; p= 0.01).

DISCUSSION

Both medical disablement figures and the amount of
musculoskeletal complaints indicate that musculoskeletal
disorders are a major work related health problem in city
busdrivers. A direct relationship is suggested between poor
ergonomics of the city buscabin and the considerable degree
of reported inconveniences regarding the physical work
environment:
- Climatological factors: 'open' working place due to the
  frequent opening of the doors.
- Vibration and forced seated position: insufficient
  adjustability of the driving seat (and other cabin
  components), no adjustable springs; vibration levels
  exceeding ISO-2631 8-hours fatigue-decreased profiency
  boundaries and, in most conditions, even exceeding
  8-hours exposure limits (Oortman Gerlings et al.,1985).

- The fourth occupational hazard (bad illumination, blinding, reflection) seems to be primarily related to night driving, bad weather conditions and neon lights.

It also is hypothesised that the shortcomings as reported in our ergonomic study and the inconveniences as reported in our survey are systematically related to (self reported) musculoskeletal disorders. The increase of these disorders until the fourth time periods in Figure 1 suggests a process of progressive deterioration of health and well-being under condition of long term exposure to workload and poor working conditions.

A plausible explanation of the decrease in the fourth time period is a health-based selection in the busdriver's population (Kompier et al., 1986), reflected in their relatively young age - compared with the Dutch working population as well as with the reference groups in Table 1 - and also in a high disablement expectation, leaving the older drivers as a small and relatively healthy selection.

NOTE [1] This article summarizes the main results of the ergonomic study. It is reported upon in more detail elsewhere (Kompier et al., 1987).

REFERENCES

Andersson, K. & Ydreborg, B., 1984. Referensdata till YMK-formulären, (Orebro).

Dijkstra, A., Grinten, M.v.d., Schlatmann, M. & Winter, C. de, 1981. Functioneren in de arbeidssituatie. (NIPG/TNO, Leiden).

Kompier, M., Meijman, T., Mulders, H. & Bullinga, R., 1986. Onderzoek naar de relatie tussen ziekteverzuim en arbeidsongeschiktheid van stadsbuschauffeurs. Tijdschrift voor Sociale Gezondheidszorg, 64, 477-480.

Kompier, M., Noord, F. van, Mulders, H. & Meijman, T., 1987. Ergonomics of the standard city buscabin, Contemporary ergonomics 1987, edited by. T. Megaw (Taylor & Francis).

Oversloot, J., Dijkstra, A., Grinten, M.v.d., Schlatmann, M. & Winter, C. de, 1982. Arbeid en gezondheid (RET) (NIPG/TNO, Leiden).

Oortman Gerlings, P., Drimmelen, D. van & Musson, Y., 1985. Trillen en schokken tijdens het werk (TU, Delft).

PHYSICAL WORK LOAD AND MUSCULOSKELETAL DISORDERS
IN THE ENGINEERING INDUSTRY

Päivi Leino & Jeddi Hasan

Department of Public Health, University of Tampere
Bix 607, SF-33101 Tampere, Finland

There exists considerable uncertainty as to the aetiological role of physical work in the development of common degenerative disorders of the musculoskeletal system (Valkenburg & Haanen 1982, Anderson 1984). Selection processes and uncontrolled factors, such as social class, create problems in interpreting the results of many epidemiological studies. Reliable measurement of load is also difficult: subjective ratings and using occupational titles as a proxy are especially problematic (Wickström 1978, Waris 1978, Hettinger 1985).

In our study 627 employees of three metal industry plants, stratified by age, sex, and occupational class, were examined in 1973 by questionnaire, interview, and clinical examination. Five years later 87 per cent of the sample were re-examined.

A physiotherapist performed the clinical examination of the musculoskeletal system, in which pains in muscles and joints were assessed by palpation, and restrictions in the movement of joints and the spine were measured. Rheumatic symptoms during the past year and chronic musculoskeletal disorders were assessed by questionnaire and interview.

An estimation of work loads was done in 1973 by observing and interviewing the subjects at the workplace, when they were performing their usual tasks. Two trained observers independently wrote down their ratings on precoded sheets, and later checked the similarity of the ratings.

Musculoskeletal morbidity as indicated by rheumatic symptoms, clinical findings, and chronic disorders, was higher in both male and female blue-collar groups than in the respective white-collar groups at baseline. Similarly, the increase in symptoms and findings, and the incidence of chronic disorders during follow-up were higher in the blue-collar groups than in the white-collar ones.

The physical work load of the blue-collar groups was higher as measured by all indices of general physical strain based on the observation (Physical Strain, Physical Load, Stereotypy, and Static Phases).

Within the occupational classes, associations between the indices of work load and those of morbidity were weak or non-existent. Physical Strain and Stereotypy showed no association with morbidity at baseline in analyses of covariance with age as covariate. In multiple regression analyses the Physical Load score (the summed lifted, carried, pushed and sustained loads) explained 3.2 % of Clinical Findings and 4.9 % of Rheumatic Symptoms in the male blue-collar group at baseline. The index of static phases explained 8.1 % of findings and 7.3 % of symptoms in the female white-collar group at baseline. No associations were observed between indices of work load at baseline and change in morbidity during follow-up.

The associations were weakened by selective movement of people with musculoskeletal disorders from heavy jobs to premature retirement and to lighter jobs prior to our baseline study.

Thus, if the gross nature of work (manual or non-manual) is accounted for, the association of musculoskeletal disorders and physical work load is low in our material. Even if selection processes are taken into account, the association seems essentially to be an ecological one, and less apparent at an individual level.

REFERENCES

Anderson, J., 1984, Arthrosis and its relation to work. Scandinavian Journal of Work, Environment & Health, 10, 429.

Hettinger, Th., 1985, Occupational hazards associated with diseases of the skeletal system. Ergonomics 28, 69

Valkenburg, H. & Haanen, H., 1982, The epidemiology of low black pain. In Symposium on idiopathic low back pain, edited by A. White & S. Gordon (The CV Mosby Company), p. 9.

Waris, P., 1979, Occupational cervicobrachial syndromes: a review. Scandinavian Journal of Work, Environment & Health, 5, suppl 3, 3.

Wickström, G., 1978, Effect of work on degenerative back disease. A review. Scandinavian Journal of Work, Environment & Health, 4, suppl 1, 1.

THE SPINAL ENGINE AND ITS GEARBOX

S. Gracovetsky and A. Carbone

Diagnospine Research Inc.
Montreal, Canada

An analysis of experimental data makes it readily apparent that the coupled motion of the spine varies greatly from one experiment to another. While some researchers have found it to be significant, others have found it to be of little importance. The coupled motion has even been found to reverse itself; that is, a lateral bend to the left may induce a clockwise as well as a counterclockwise axial rotation. It is an accepted fact that the spine moves synchronously with the pelvis during walking. We also know that we can move the spine without any pelvic involvement when executing a lateral bend.

Quite clearly the spine does not behave as a simple flexible rod. If it did, a lateral bend with lordosis would always result in a specific axial rotation. The spine, however, exhibits more complex responses to mechanical inputs. We have hypothesised that the basic difference between a flexible rod and the spine lies in the construction of the facet joints.

To appreciate and understand the effect of the facets on the coupled motion of the spine, we analysed the conditions under which the facets would make contact during a lateral bend.

In the first simplified analysis, the problem is reduced to the representation shown in Figure 1(a). Here the subchrondral plates of the facets are modelled as short segments separated by the thickness of the cartilage. The entire intervertebral joint is assumed to rotate around an axis perpendicular to the plane of the figure that intersects the plane. In this example, the angle of rotation has been set at 5° to the left. Figure 1(b) shows the resultant locations of V_1 and V_2 corresponding to a 5° left-hand lateral rotation of the upper vertebrae V_1 vis-à-vis V_2. The centre of rotation is denoted as CR. The disc motion is abnormal, thus indicating that a rotation around that particular centre of rotation is not physiological.

Figure 1(c) illustrates a possible rotation around CR. The variation in cartilage thickness occurring during the change in the relative position of the facet is inconsequential to the logic of the argument. Facet contact may be defined as either a bone-to-bone contact or that which occurs when the two subchrondral plates are separated by a given thickness of cartilage. In the latter case, contact will be considered to have occurred earlier, without affecting our conclusions.

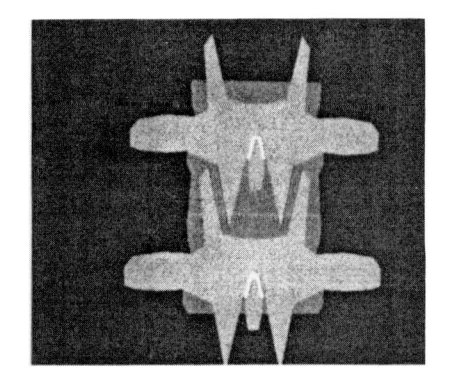

Definition : V_1 = Upper vertebrae
V_2 = Lower vertebrae
Figure 1(a)

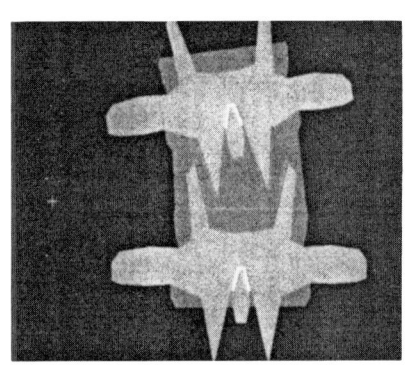

Definition CR is indicated by a +
Figure 1(b)

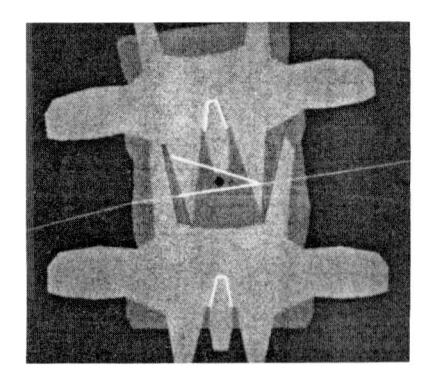

Rotation around CR indicated by a dot
Figure 1(c)

A question therefore arises. Can one find a location for the centre of rotation (CR) so that the left facet contacts? In fact, we can select a contact point on the left facet and calculate the corresponding locus of all the centres of rotation (LFL). We can repeat the same process for the right facet. The results of the calculation of these loci are outlined in Figure 2.

Therefore, whenever the CR is located anywhere on the lower locus, a 5° lateral bend to the left results in the transmission of compressive forces through the facet. When viewed from above, the V_2 vertebra rotates in a clockwise direction.

Similarly, when the CR is located on the upper locus (RFL), the right facet will be set under compression for the same 5° lateral bend to the left. This case is the opposite of the earlier one. It will result in the counterclockwise rotation of the lower V_2 vertebra, as viewed from above.

One should note that the loci of LFL and RFL intersect (Figure 2(c)). At that particular point, the centre of rotation is such that the right and left facets are simultaneously compressed because the CR is on RFL and LFL simultaneously. Hence, the V_2 vertebra is locked and cannot rotate. This phenomenon occurs during physical exercises in which the spine is bent laterally without any pelvic axial rotation. It also demonstrates the importance of precise control of the location of the centre of rotation. A relatively minor displacement of the position of CR can switch it from one locus to the other and therefore reverse or stop the rotation of V_2 and, consequently, the pelvic rotation.

We can now appreciate the variations between earlier experimental analyses of the coupled motion of the spine. In the past, the general lack of appreciation of the importance of controlling the position of the centre of rotation has made the experimental outcome totally dependent upon the particular mechanical configuration of the set-up in which these *in vitro* measurements were made. Our simple model also gives us clues to a possible explanation for the loss of disc space and facet tropism.

The loss of disc space is generally perceived as being an unavoidable consequence of some form of disc degeneration, regardless of whether this degeneration is caused by repeated injury or some other process. The equations of the loci indicate that they depend upon the disc height. As disc space decreases, the RFL and LRL move closer to the centre.

This finding suggests that, even if, for any reason (e.g. injury of the disc), the centre of rotation (CR) should be unable to move as freely as before, it will still be possible to maintain appropriate facet contact (and, hence, normal gait). In this case, as the disc loses height, the loci shift toward CR. So, in the event of injury, a loss of disc space should not necessarily be looked upon as an aggravating factor.

There may, however, also be some other mechanism resulting in a similar compensatory action as the equation of the loci also depends upon the facet's angle of

28   Musculoskeletal disorders at work

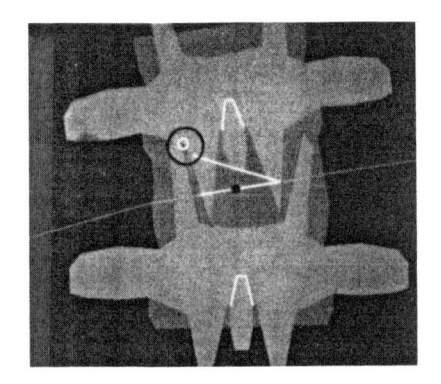

The Left facet contacts when V_1 is rotated to the left around CR. The contact occurs when CR is anywhere on the corresponding locus. Here, the lower vetebra is driven in a clockwise axial rotation.

Figure 2(a)

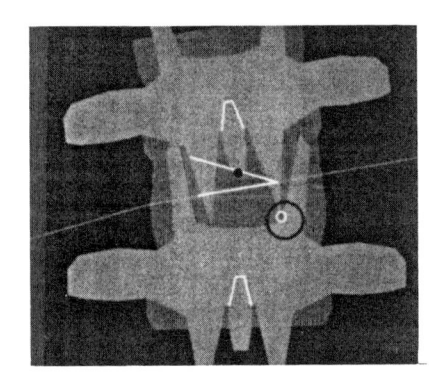

The Right facet contacts when V1 is rotated to the left around CR. This is the opposite of above. The contact occurs when CR is anywhere on its corresponding locus. Here the lower vertebrae is driven in a counter clockwise axial rotation.

Figure 2(b)

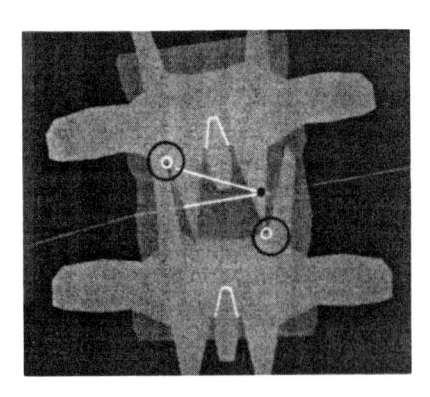

Here both facets are compресsѕed simultaneously, and there is no facet contact. Where CR lies at the intersection of both loci, we have simultaneously left and right facet contacting. No axial rotation is possible.

Figure 2(c)

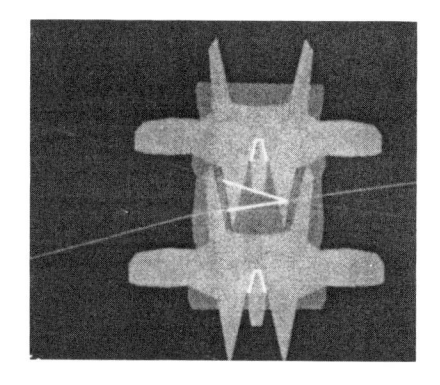

Normal position showing the two loci.

Figure 3(a)

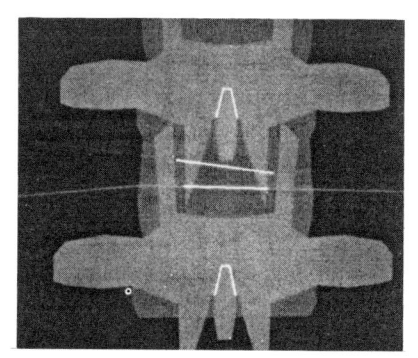

The facets are remodelled and are almost parallel. Note the displacement of the loci. Compare with 3(a) above.

Figure 3(b)

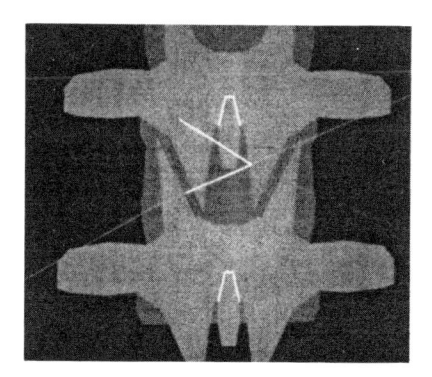

The facet angle is opened and the shift in loci position is evident

Figure 3(c)

inclination from the vertical position. When this facet angle is modified, the corresponding loci are shifted. (Fig. 3) Facet remodelling has essentially the same effect on the loci of the centre of rotation as a loss of disc height.

We would like to suggest that facet tropism ought to be viewed as a compensatory mechanism which, in conjunction with a loss of disc height, permits a damaged joint to maintain the appropriate facet involvement during locomotion. In fact, it is difficult to conceive of bone remodelling (as extensive as that sometimes seen in CT scans) without the presence of a continuous source of mechanical excitation. As bone responds to stress, we can hypothesise that it is the regular, alternating pounding of the facets, ensuring the transmission of forces sufficient to drive the pelvis, that is responsible for this remodelling.

COMPUTER-AIDED ANALYSIS OF TRUNK AND SHOULDER POSTURE

W. M. Keyserling, Ph.D.
L. J. Fine, M.D.
L. Punnett, Sc.D.

Center for Ergonomics
The University of Michigan
1205 Beal Avenue
Ann Arbor, Michigan 48109 USA

INTRODUCTION

Awkward posture of the trunk and shoulders can be caused by several factors in the workplace, including: poor work station layout, inappropriate design or selection of equipment and hand tools, incorrect work methods, and/or the anthropometric characteristics of the worker. In some situations, the interaction of one or more of these factors can contribute to awkward posture. For example, if the height of an assembly bench has been properly adjusted to comfortably accommodate a small worker (e.g., a 5th percentile female), it may create excessive trunk flexion for a large worker (e.g., a 95th percentile male). On the other hand, if the height of an overhead conveyor has been adjusted to provide head clearance for a large male, it may create excessive shoulder abduction for a smaller person. If not controlled, awkward postures can cause fatigue and contribute to the development of musculoskeletal disorders. This is of particular concern on highly repetitive jobs due to the frequency of awkward posture and the cumulative effects of exposure (Corlett, et al., 1979, Grandjean, 1980).

A new computer-aided system for posture analysis has been developed in conjunction with an epidemiologic study of occupational trunk and shoulder disorders. (See: Fine, et al., 1987; and Punnett, et al., 1987.) In developing this system, it was desirable to include the following features:
- <u>Conceptually Simple</u> -- The posture classification system should be easily understood, learned, and used by persons who are not experts in ergonomics.
- <u>Non-invasive</u> -- Data collection procedures should require minimal interference with the subject's work. Specifically, the system should not require that any hardware be attached to the subject's body.

- Time-efficient -- Data collection and reduction procedures should be sufficiently time-efficient to permit the evaluation of a large number of jobs with reasonable human resources. Specifically, less than 30 minutes should be required to collect and reduce data for a short-cycle (approximately 75 seconds) job.
- Continuous and Complete Record -- The system should produce an uninterrupted record of postural activity for the entire job. Furthermore, it should be feasible to superimpose the results of the posture analysis and a task analysis on the same time scale.
- Ergonomically Relevant -- The system should identify work postures and associated tasks that are associated with increased risk of fatigue or musculoskeletal disorders.

METHOD

Posture Classification System

The classification system presented in Figure 1 defines a menu of standard positions of the trunk and shoulders. This menu was developed by observing videotapes of a wide variety of work activities to establish a taxonomy of common work postures. (Keyserling, 1986a). Conceptually, this classification scheme is similar to those used in the OWAS (Karhu, et. al., 1977) and VIRA (Kilbom, et al., 1985) systems.

The trunk is considered to be in a neutral posture if it remains within 20 degrees of the vertical and if axial twisting is limited to no more than 20 degrees. Non-neutral standard postures include: extension (bending backwards), mild flexion (bending forward 20-45 degrees), severe flexion (bending forward more than 45 degrees), lateral bending, and twisting. These categories can be used to describe a subject who is either standing or sitting. A special category exists for workers who must lie on their side or back.

Shoulder posture is determined by the included angle between the trunk and the humerus. The shoulder is considered to be in a neutral posture if this angle is less than 45 degrees. Non-neutral postures include: mild flexion/abduction (an included angle of 45-90 degrees) and severe flexion/abduction (an included angle of more than 90 degrees). The system does not consider the bearing of the humerus when classifying shoulder posture.

Data Collection and Reduction

Data collection procedures are similar to time study methods developed by industrial engineers. The goals of a time study are to document the sequence of tasks required to

CLASSIFYING TRUNK POSTURE

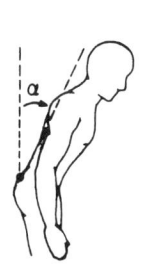

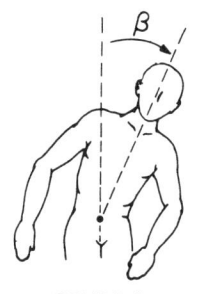

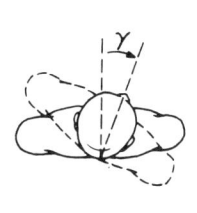

FLEXION/EXTENSION
α measured in the sagittal plane

BENDING
β measured in the frontal plane

TWISTING
γ is rotation about the long axis of the trunk

NEUTRAL occurs when the trunk is within 20 degrees of the vertical with less than 20 degrees of twisting

STANDARD TRUNK POSTURES	
1. Stand-Extension ($\alpha < -20°$)	6. Lie-On Back or Side
2. Stand-Neutral	7. Sit-Neutral
3. Stand-Mild Flexion ($20° < \alpha \leq 45°$)	8. Sit-Mild Flexion
4. Stand-Severe Flexion ($\alpha > 45°$)	9. Sit-Twisted/Bent
5. Stand-Twisted/Bent (β or $\gamma > 20°$)	

CLASSIFYING SHOULDER POSTURE

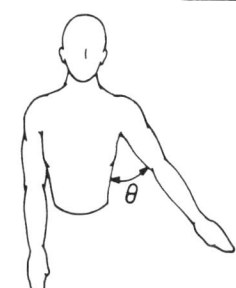

SHOULDER FLEXION/ABDUCTION is the included angle θ between the trunk and the humerus.
NEUTRAL occurs when θ is less than 45 degrees.

STANDARD SHOULDER POSTURES
1. Neutral ($\theta \leq 45°$)
2. Mild Flexion/Abduction ($45° < \theta \leq 90°$)
3. Severe Flexion/Abduction ($\theta > 90°$)

Figure 1. Standard postures of the trunk and shoulders (Keyserling, 1986a.)

perform a job and to measure the time required to perform each task. The goals of posture analysis are to document patterns of postural activity at the trunk and shoulders and to measure the amount of time spent in each standard posture.

The first step in posture analysis is to produce a videotape of the job of interest. If job redesign is a desired outcome of the analysis, workstation dimensions (bench heights, reach distances, handtool dimensions, etc.) should be measured and a sequential task description should be prepared at the same time that the videotape is produced (Keyserling, 1986b). If the resulting data are to be used strictly for epidemiologic studies, it is not necessary to obtain these data.

The second step in posture analysis is to extract postural data from the videotape. To do this, the tape is played back at the same speed at which it was recorded. An analyst views the tape and classifies trunk and shoulder postures using the standard categories depicted in Figure 1. As the tape is played, a personal computer is used for time keeping and data logging. (This permits the analyst to devote uninterrupted attention to the videotape.) Each of the standard postures is assigned a key on the computer. Whenever the worker changes posture, the analyst strikes the key corresponding to the new posture. The value of the new posture and the time of the posture change are recorded by the computer and stored on diskette for subsequent analysis and archiving (Keyserling, 1986a).

To eliminate the need to observe multiple joints simultaneously, the tape must be played one time for each joint of interest. (Even experienced analysts report extreme difficulty in tracking multiple joints.) Because the same video frame is used as the starting time for each analysis, the postural activity of multiple joints can be superimposed on a common time scale. This feature is useful in recreating composite postures of the trunk and shoulders at any point during the work cycle.

Data Analysis and Interpretation

Upon completion of data entry, the system produces two reports for each body joint: 1) a statistical summary of postural activity at the joint, and 2) a graphical description of all postural states and changes.

The summary report includes the following descriptive statistics for each joint:
- The frequency per basic job cycle that each standard posture is entered.
- The total time per job cycle and the time fraction of the job cycle spent in each standard posture.
- Minimum, maximum, and mean times spent in each standard posture.
- The frequency of posture changes during the job cycle and the mean time between posture changes.
- The duration of the basic job cycle.

The summary report provides a good "snapshot" description of the postural attributes of a job, and can be used to rank order a list of jobs based on relative levels of postural stress. The descriptive statistics can be used to develop dose indices for epidemiologic studies of posture-related musculoskeletal disorders (see Punnett, et al., 1987; and Fine, et al., 1987).

The descriptive statistics can also be used to develop estimates of biomechanical stresses. For example, trunk flexion in the sagittal plane increases the compressive forces acting at the L5/S1 intervertebral disc (Chaffin and Andersson, 1984). Table 1 presents estimated spinal compression values for selected trunk flexion angles. (These angles include the midpoints and "break" points of the standard trunk flexion postures presented in Figure 1. Two conditions are considered: 1) no load held in the hands, and 2) a load of 100 N held in the sagittal plane.) Maximum Spinal Compression (MSC) for the work cycle corresponds to the posture-load combination associated with the highest value in Table 1. An estimate of cumulative spinal compression can be developed by computing:

$$CSC = \sum T_i \times SC_i$$

where:
CSC = cumulative spinal compression (N-sec),
T_i = time spent in posture i (sec),
SC_i = spinal compression in posture i (N), and
n = number of different standard postures.

Work is currently underway to determine if MSC and/or CSC are significant factors in the development of trunk disorders.

The graphical description of postural activity (the second report produced by the posture analysis system) is a valuable tool for evaluating a job to identify specific causes of postural stress. By plotting major job tasks and postures of the trunk and shoulders on a common time scale, it is possible to identify specific work activities responsible for high levels of postural stress. Additional information on these procedures is available elsewhere (Keyserling, 1986b.)

SYSTEM PERFORMANCE AND DISCUSSION

The posture analysis system described above has been used to generate exposure data for a study of automobile assembly workers (see Fine, et al., 1987; Punnett, et al., 1987). Operating experience with the system has shown that a trained analyst can evaluate a short-cycle (60-75 sec) job in about 20 min. Results obtained with the system are repeatable and compare favorably with results obtained using a "freeze-frame" technique (Keyserling, 1986a).

ACKNOWLEDGEMENT

This research was supported in part through a research contract with the Ford Motor Company (Body and Assembly Operations).

Table I. Estimated spinal compression forces (N) for selected trunk postures and loads. (Estimates based on 50th percentile male anthropometry using the Univ. of Michigan two-dimensional strength model, Chaffin and Andersson, 1984.)

Trunk Flexion Angle (deg.)	Spinal Compression (N)			
	No Load Force	%AL*	100 N Load Force	%AL*
0	285	8.3	366	10.7
10	783	22.8	1012	29.5
20	1207	35.2	1550	45.2
33.5	1672	48.7	2127	62.0
45	1939	56.5	2454	71.5
67.5	2257	65.8	2858	83.3
90	2278	66.4	2922	85.2

* Percentage of NIOSH (1981) Action Limit.

REFERENCES

Chaffin, D. & Andersson, G., 1984, Occupational Biomechanics, (New York: Wiley-Interscience).

Corlett, E., Madeley, S. & Manenica, I., 1979, Ergonomics, 22, 357.

Fine, L., Punnett, L. & Keyserling, W., 1987, An epidemiological study of postural risk factors for shoulder disorders in industry. In Proceedings: Musculoskeletal Disorders at Work, edited by P. Buckle (London, Taylor & Francis).

Grandjean, E., 1980, Fitting the Task to the Man, (London: Taylor & Francis, Ltd.).

Karhu, O., Kansi, P., and Kuorinka, I., 1977, Applied Ergonomics, 8, 199.

Keyserling, W., 1986a, Ergonomics, 29, 569.

Keyserling, W., 1986b, American Industrial Hygiene Association Journal, 47, 641.

Kilbom, A. Persson, J. and Jonsson, B., 1985, Risk factors for work-related disorders of the neck and shoulder -- with special emphasis on working postures and movements. In Proceedings: International Symposium on the Ergonomics of Working Posture (Zadar, Yugoslavia).

NIOSH, 1981, Work Practices Guide for Manual Lifting, (Cincinnati, NIOSH).

Punnett, L., Fine, L. & Keyserling, W., 1987, An epidemiological study of postural risk factors for back disorders in industry. In Proceedings: Musculoskeletal Disorders at Work, edited by P. Buckle (London, Taylor & Francis).

ARM-LIFT STRENGTH VARIATION DUE TO TASK PARAMETERS

SHRAWAN KUMAR

Department of Physical Therapy, University of
Alberta Edmonton, Alberta T6G 2G4, Canada

INTRODUCTION

A number of authors have reported an association between the physical stress of the job and low back pain occurrence. In a longitudinal study of low-back pain Chaffin Park (1973) reported that the incidence rate of low-back pain was correlated with higher lifting strength requirements. Based on this conclusion Chaffin et al (1978) investigated the relationship between the pre-employment strength characteristics of 551 employees in six plants and the incidence and severity of back problems over a period of 18 months. They found that the workers likelyhood of sustaining back injury significantly increased (3:1) when the severity of the job approached or exceeded the demonstrated isometric strength of the workers in standardised postures. However, the validity of static measures has come under question (Kroemer 1984). The important objection has been the lack of applicability of static measures to predominantly dynamic industrial situations.

Kumar & Chaffin (1985) and Kumar et al (1986) have reported isometric and isokinetic arm lift strength in young adults between knuckle to shoulder heights at three different lifting velocities. They reported an inverse relationship between strength capabilitiy and the velocity of lift. All tests reported by them were performed at a preselected reach distance which was fixed throughout the test. The effect of variation of reach distance of the task on strength characteristics have not been reported. therefore a study was designed to measure the isometric and isokinetic strength with changing task parameters.

METHODOLOGY

Testing equipment and measurement: For strength testing a specially designed and fabricated piece of equipment was used. For a complete description of this machine the reader is referred to Kumar et al (1985) and Kumar et al (1986). However the salient features of this instrument are as follows. This Dynamic Strength Tester was designed to perform a two handed isometric or isokenetic lift. The handle bar of this strength tester could be adjusted to any height for isometric test. For isokinetic test it provided a constant speed motion regardless of applied force. The speed of motion could be adjusted using servo control mechanism. The constant velocity was achieved by coupling the handle bar through a non-stretchable canvas strap and a one-way clutch to a shaft rotating at fixed pre-set speed. The clutch uncoupled the mechanical resistance of the motor driven system until the threshold speed was reached. This allowed a resistance free movement of the handlebar below the pre-set speed When the speed threshold was reached the clutch engaged the constant speed shaft and controlled the speed with high resistance. The force applied on the handle was measured by a load cell (Interface Model SM 500-500 lb.) which was inserted between the handle bar and the canvas strap. The output of the load cell was fed to a HP 9826 computer through a force monitor (ST-1) and data acquisition system (HP 3054 A) with an A to D converter. A displacement potentiometer was used to measure the displacement of the handle bar and its output similarly processed and fed to the computer. A customised software was developed to acquire and log data at 50 Hz. Isometric and isokinetic strength values were also normalized against the standard posture arm lift peak strength.

Subjects and Tasks: Eleven normal males with a mean age of 22.5 years, a mean weight of 73.3 kg. and a mean height of 177.6 cm. and ten normal females with a mean age of 22.3 years, a mean weight of 58.5 kg. and a mean height of 162.7 cm. without any back disorder volunteered for the study. These subjects were asked to perform isokinetic lifts in upright standing posture from knuckle height to shoulder height in a sagittally symmetrical plane at half reach, three quarters reach and full reach distances. The individual reach distance of every subject was measured from the acromian process to the centre of the grip with a 90^0 flexed shoulder joint and straight arm. The worksite was marked at full reach distance from the centre of the lifting handle in sagittal plane. Three quarters and half of this distance was marked from the centre of the handle bar to represent three quarters and half reach of the subject.

The subjects were asked to heel the randomly preselected reach line and perform the lift exerting their maximal effort throughout the range of motion without jerking. Every subject was given identical familiarisation session and instruction. The lifts were begun at 10 cm. below the knuckle height and terminated past the shoulder height. The data was, however, collected from knuckle height to shoulder height only. For isometric tests the initial position of isokinetic test was chosen as the test position. The subjects were also tested in the standard posture arm lift (Chaffin et al 1978) for isometric strength.

Data Analysis: The peak strengths of males and females in isometric and isokinetic conditions were obtained and normalised against standard posture arm lift peak strength and compared. These values were also subjected to one-way analysis of variance for the effect of reach. A Newman-Keuls post hoc test and a correlation analysis between the strength value and reach distance of the task was done.

RESULT AND DISCUSSION

The isometric as well as isokinetic strengths of males were significantly higher than those of females (Figure 1).

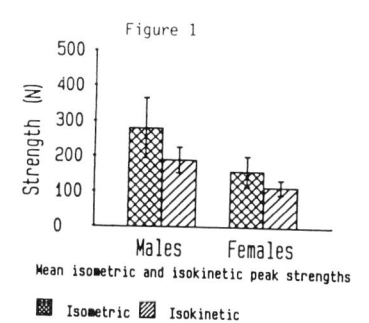

Figure 1
Mean isometric and isokinetic peak strengths
■ Isometric ▨ Isokinetic

The female's arm lift strength ranged between 48.5% to 69.2% The standard posture isometric and half reach isometric strengths of female subjects were 51% and 48.5%

of male population. Three quarters and full reach isometric as well as isokinetic arm strengths of females ranged between 63% to 69%.

The isometric strength was invariably significantly higher than that of isokinetic strength ($p < 0.001$, Figure 1).

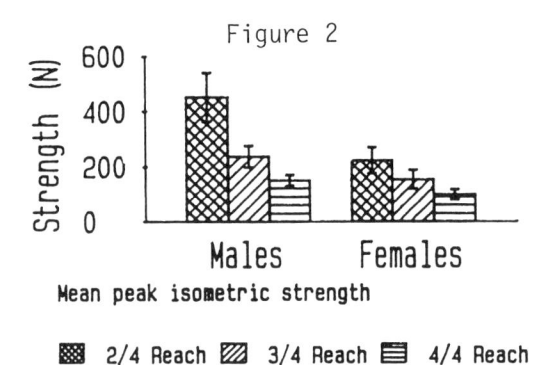

Figure 2

Mean peak isometric strength

▓ 2/4 Reach ▨ 3/4 Reach ☰ 4/4 Reach

Both isometric as well as isokinetic strength was found to be inversely related to the reach distance (Figures 2 and 3). The quantative relationship is exhibited in the negative correlation coefficients (Table 1).

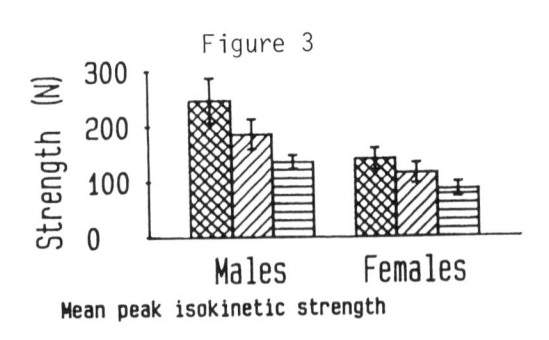

Figure 3

Mean peak isokinetic strength

▓ 2/4 Reach ▨ 3/4 Reach ☰ 4/4 Reach

Table 1. The correlation coefficients of the strength and reach.

Gender	Condition	Correlation Coefficient	Probability
Male	Isometric	-.76	.01
	Isokinetic	-.69	.01
Female	Isometric	-.63	.01
	Isokinetic	-.67	.01

The standard posture peak strength for males and females were observed to be 310 N and 158 N respectively. The relative magnitude of isometric and isokinetic strength with increasing reach distance normalised against the standard posture peak strength is given in Table 2.

One-way analysis of variance carried out revealed a significant effect of reach distance on the strength observed (p < 0.001). A Newman-Keul's multiple comparison established that the three reach distances were uniquely different in their effect on strength.

Table 2. Relative magnitude of strength expressed as per cent of standard posture peak isometric strength.

	Isometric			Isokinetic		
Gender	2/4 Reach	3/4 Reach	4/4 Reach	2/4 Reach	3/4 Reach	4/4 Reach
Male	166	85	52	93	68	46
Female	144	107	66	107	85	62

Since the most jobs carried out in the industry are not in static mode and are performed at different reach distances away from the body the isokinetic strength measured at standardised distances may be valuable in designing tasks. The current study clearly demonstrates that the strength characteristics are subject to significant variation when conditions change from isometric to isokinetic mode or when the effort lever arm is altered. Increasing the velocity of movement causes a further reduction in strength (Kumar & Chaffin 1985 and Kumar et al 1986). Based on these findings it is suggested that the dynamic strength measures be incorporated in job design considerations.

References

Chaffin, D.B., Herrin, G.D. and Keyserling W.M. (1978) Preemployment strength testing. An updated position. *Journal of Occupational Medicine*, 20, 403-408

Chaffin, D.B. and Park, K.S. (1973) A longitudinal study of low-back pain as associated with occuational weight lifting factors. *American Industrial Hygiene Association Journal*, 34, 513-525

Kroemer, K.H.E. (1984) Ergonomics of manual materials handling. A review of models, methods and techniques. *Proceedings of the 1984 International Conference on Occupational Ergonomics.* 56-60 Kumar, S. and Chaffin, D.B. (1985) Static and dynamic listing strengths of young males. In *Biomechanics X*. Editor B. Jonsson. Human Kinetics. In press.

Kumar, S., Chaffin, D.B. and Foulke, J. (1985) Methodology for the measurement of dynamic lifting strength In *Biomechanics X*, Editor B. Jonsson. Human Kinetics. In press.

Kumar, S., Chaffin, D.B. and Redfern, M. (1986) Isometric and isokinetic back and arm lifting strengths: Device and Measurement. Manuscript submitted to *Journal of Biomechanics*.

PORTABLE MICROCOMPUTER BASED TECHNIQUE FOR POSTURE OR
ACTIVITY RECORDING IN THE FIELD

A.G. Clark*, K. Browne**, R. Madeley** and J.E. Ridd*

* Ergonomics Research Unit, Robens Institute, and
** Psychology Department, University of Surrey,
Guildford, Surrey

This paper describes a menu driven portable microcomputer program adapted for the Epson PX-8, to assist in posture or activity data aquisition in the field. It features the facility to store data in files on RAM disc or on microcassettes driven from a unit on the machine. Data files can be transferred through an RS232 port to a main frame computer where existing Fortran programs can be used to convert them into a form suitable for analysis using statistical packages such as SPSSX. Initial laboratory validation studies of the method were conducted over a 5 day period. On day 5 a mean accuracy of **92.3%**(SD 2.5) correct key strikes was achieved. Trials are being carried out to determine whether this level of accuracy can be maintained in field situations and whether training will significantly improve this level of accuracy.

Introduction

Target groups at risk of musculoskeletal disorders can be identified from epidemiological surveys and further studies undertaken at the site of work to more thoroughly investigate probable links between the nature of work and the associated risk. Hence, there is a need for a thoroughly validated technique to collect reliable information about the typical activities that are undertaken at work, their frequencies within a shift, durations, and the body postures associated with them, as well the worker tolerance of them.

There are a number of techniques for the collection of this kind of information and these have been reviewed recently by Colombini (1985). She concludes that there is a case for using methods in combination coupled with epidemiological studies of the main health problems associated with postural stress, and further that the main problem awaiting solution is the criteria for interpreting the data.

The portable microcomputer has the potential to automate the direct recording of behavioural events for both field and laboratory work. This paper reports on the development, reliability, and validity of a menu driven program adapted from software first developed for the Epson HX-20 as a means of recording animal and human behaviour in their natural habitat, (Browne and Madeley 1983). The software has been adapted to assist in the detailed acquisition of data concerned with human postures and activities in the work place, on the Epson PX-8 and complies with the main criteria identified by Corlett (1979), for an effective method for describing working postures.

The PX-8 portable microcomputer is a battery-powered, 64 kilobytes RAM machine with a built in microcassette drive and 80 characters x 8 lines LCD screen. Together with a full sized QWERTY keyboard it is small enough to rest in the lap of the seated observer or be carried on a waist high tray supported from straps. The program is suitable for an observer unfamiliar with computers and affords the capacity to read up to one observation per second with minimum keyboard input.

Data files can be stored on RAM or microcassette and later transferred from them to a main frame computer where existing Fortran programs can be used to convert them into a form suitable for analysis using statistical packages such as SPSSX or SAS.

Description of the Program

The menu driven program allows the operator to choose one of six main sub-programs. a) Library, b) Observation c) Data Retrieval, d) Quit Package, e) File management, f) Frequencies.

a) The Library sub-program provides facilities to create, amend, store or print libraries of two types; one for selected postures and activities and the other for selected subjects and devices, relevent to the job under observation. Each descriptive entry into the library associates a single alphabetic key with a posture or activity and a single numeric key with a subject or a device. Thus during an ´observation´ postures and/or activities may be associated with subjects and/or devices by striking the relevent keys on the QWERTY keyboard in sequence.

b) ´Observations´ is the event recording process and uses the current ´library´ to associate single key depression with pre-defined descriptors. A valid ´library´ must have been created or loaded prior to using the ´Observation´ program. During operation the sequence of events is conserved and each key depression presented on the LCD screen in the form of its descriptor. The elapsed time from the start of an observation is automatically recorded alongside each descriptor.

There are three types of observation possible with this program: (i) Single subject recordings that associate one particular subject or device with a number of postures and activities; (ii) Multi-subject recordings that associate two or more subjects or devices with a number of postures and activities. (iii) Interactive recordings that associate the postures and activities that occur between subjects and devices.

Postures and activities can be recorded consecutively or concurrently and error messages are set up with respect to each mode. Once the observation type and mode have been selected, the user enters a sample identification and test number before starting the event recording session.

c) Following an ´Observation´ the researcher uses the ´Data Retrieval´ program to output the data on to a portable printer (Epson P40). The recorded data is in a readable format that can be readily examined. In addition, the data may be copied on to micro cassette tape, RAM disc or floppy Disc (Epson PF10) for transfer to a larger computer and later statistical analyses.

d), e) and f) will not be described, since they are not directly involved with the capture of data.

The experiment described here assesses the ability of an operator to accurately strike labeled keys on a micro computer keyboard when cued from a VDU screen with the words that appear on the keyboard labels.

This approach was adopted as a first step, in favour of showing subjects video recordings of activities, since this would require that subjects were trained prior to the experiment to chose unambiguously the definitions of the displayed events.

Subjects

Ten subjects, 8 males and 2 females took part in the experiment. All had previous experience in using keyboards, and 3 could touch type, two of whom were female). None had any visual impairment that was not correctable with spectacles.

Method

The subjects were seated in front of a BBC B+ VDU which was programmed to present cue words in a random sequence on the screen at time intervals selected randomly from a range (0.5 to 2.5 secs between each change of word) representative of posture elements of digging a hole, for a period of five minutes.

The test was run on five consecutive days. On the first day the test duration was two minutes in order to familiarise the operators with the experimental apparatus. On the subsequent four days the experimental time was five minutes. The BBC B+ was programmed to file the order and exact time that the cue words were presented on the screen. At the same time the Epson PX-8 program (Posturegram) was similarly filing the sequence of key strikes and time of key strike of each of the subjects responses to cues from the BBC B+.

In order to compare responses between subjects within a day, the order of presentation of cues and the time interval between each cue was the same for each subject. Having been created randomly at the start of each day a file of the sequence and timing was stored and available for presentation to each subject.

Direct comparisons were made between the records from the BBC B+ and the Epson PX-8 to calculate the percentage correct key strikes per session. Analysis of variance was performed to test for significance in differences between subjects and between days.

Results

The figure shows the relationship between time (days) and number of correct key hits minus wrongly struck keys and erroneously struck keys, represented as a percentage of the number of displayed cue words.

The mean (SD) percentage of correct key strikes from days 2 to 5 were 82.4 (5.8), 89.9 (2.0), 88.9 (4.3), and 90.0 (2.8) respectively.

The results of the analysis of variance show a significant (p<0.001), rise in correct key hits with day of the experiment but that the difference between the subjects in accuracy of hitting keys was insignificant.

Figure to show percentage correct key strikes over 5 days.
       Day 1; familiarisation for 2 minutes.
       Days 2-5; 5 minutes per day.
       Symbols represent individual subjects.

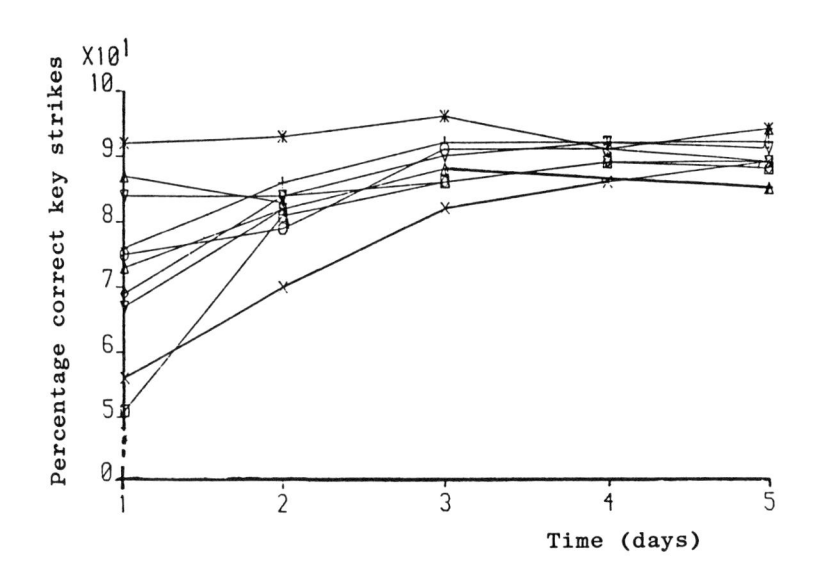

Discussion

The significant rise in accuracy in observation of cue words but lack of significant difference between subjects reveals a need for training in using the technique but that a high level of inter-subject reliability can be expected for non ambiguous cues. In order to maintain this high level of inter-subject (ie. inter-observer) reliability for data collection there is a need to catagorise postures or activities accurately and with little room for misinterpretation. Raty (1985) demonstrated the pertinence of this in their test of inter-observer reliability of direct observation. They used posture charts for recording the data and accepted levels of agreement between observers of no less than 75%. They discovered that only observation in the catagories of bend, stand, walk, kneel, sit and squat were reliable. The posture categories push, pull, lift, brace, carry, reach and twist were below this level. The postures, however, had not been defined closely, consequently lift could be used by the observer to define any posture that resulted in raising an object with the hands, likewise twist could be used to define any movement of the shoulders relative to the pelvis. What one observer in a pair might consider to be a lift or twist the other may ignore. The training of observers to use categories within more tightly defined parameters would help to improve concurrence.

Trials are being carried out to determine whether this level of accuracy can be maintained in field situations and whether training will further improve this level of accuracy. Inter-observer reliability is also being tested. As with all event recording devices that rely on human input, interpretation of the event under study may vary between operators unless a strict code of operation is followed which may require special training and prudent library creation to ensure the successful use of the system.

Conclusions

1) The 'Posturegram' software run on the Epson PX-8 offers an easy to operate, and flexible method of collecting posture and activity information in the field.

2) Data files can be transferred easily to a more powerful computer for statistical analysis, although this does not solve the problem of how to interpret the data.

3) High levels of accuracy can be achieved in operators observing non ambiguous cues.

References

Baty, D., Buckle, P.W., and Stubbs, D.A., 1986, Egonomics of working postures; models and methods. Taylor and Francis.
Browne, K.D., and Madeley, R. 1985, ´Ethogram´ -an event recording package. Journal of Child Psychology and Psychiatry,26,6, Software Survey Section, P.III.
Colombini,D., Occhipinti,E., Molteni,G., Grieco,A., Pedotti, A., Boccardi, S., Frigo, C. and Menoni, O.,1985, Posture Analysis. Ergonomics,28,1,275-284.
Corlett, E.N., Madeley, S.J., and Manenica, I.,1979, Posture targetting:a Technique for Recording Working Postures. Ergonomics,22,3,357-366.

EVALUATION OF WORK POSTURES
I. A model for evaluation of seated work tasks

Jörgen A. E. Eklund (+), Stefan Zettergren (*),
Per Odenrick (+)

(+) Department of Industrial Ergonomics,
   University of Linköping,
   S-581 83 Linköping, SWEDEN

(*) Occupational Health Center,
   Swedish Steel Corporation (SSAB),
   Box 1000, S-613 01 Oxelösund, SWEDEN

INTRODUCTION

High frequencies of musculoskeletal problems have been reported from several seated work tasks. Examples of such tasks are sewing machine operation, assembly in the electronics industry, and vehicle driving. Some of the tasks involve high muscle load, and others repetitive loadings. Also, constrained postures often appear. In order to facilitate the analysis of seated work tasks, a model for evaluation of these tasks has been proposed. By understanding how influences from the work are related to the responses and effects on the sitter, and to the workplace and chair design, it becomes possible to control and manipulate design in order to minimize adverse effects. In this way, the appropriateness of the work station can be improved by using a systematic analysis of the most important work factors rather than by using empirical attempts. In this respect, the concept of effective design can be defined as a design which causes a minimum of adverse effects.

THE MODEL

The model incorporates and describes characteristics, such as demands and restrictions of the work (see Table 1). These demands and restrictions of the task and the workplace should be seen as objective descriptions, defining the performance of the task and the characteristics of the workplace. One example of a restriction is limited space. Furthermore, the model includes responses and effects on the sitter, and these may be initial or subsequent.

Table 1. A model for evaluation of seated work tasks.

DEMANDS AND RESTRICTIONS	RESPONSES AND EFFECTS	
	INITIAL	SUBSEQUENT
Work task Positions required (hands, arms, back) Movements required Force required (magnitude, direction) Precision required Time restrictions (frequency, duration) Space restrictions **Workplace** Size Height Distance Angle Object Aids Space and movement restrictions Acceleration forces Visibility Light Environmental influences **Individual** Anthropometry Capacity Psychological state	Postures (back, neck, arms, trunk, legs) Loads (back, neck, shoulders, arms, legs) Pressure (inner organs, skin) Influence upon the blood flow Discomfort	Discomfort Pain Disease Reduction in performance
Measures	**Measures**	**Measures**
Workplace dimensions Work weights Work forces Work reaches Work time patterns Anthropometry Strength	Biomechanical load EMG Body height shrinkage Rating scales Dilation of body parts Linear measurements Posture	Rating scales Clinical examinations Epidemiological studies

The model shows how the initial responses and effects can be used as indicators of the appropriateness of the task, seat and workplace design. Such an approach in the evaluation process has many advantages. A number of methods for measurement already exist. The responses and effects can also be measured and assessed immediately, which is a major advantage in applied design evaluations. Looking to the initial responses and effects allows preventive measures to be taken in the stage before the adverse effects occur. The subsequent responses and effects are more long-term in their manifestation and may be more difficult to measure. Experimental laboratory studies using subsequent responses and effects are in principle impossible.

One of the major task influences on the postures chosen and the loads imposed upon the sitter is the visual demand. In many cases, the ability to see the work object is absolutely essential. The worker often has to adopt one viewing angle for long periods of time, and sometimes also a certain eye position. These factors are often explained through task analysis. The distance between the eye and the work object can, for example, be determined by the size of the work object, the contrast and the lighting. In some tasks, the degree of postural freedom is heavily restricted due to the visual demands, in the worst case allowing only one head, upper limb and trunk posture, e.g. in microscope use.

Another major task influence is the demand on hand manipulation. In order to perform the physical aspects of the task, certain actions or operations must be conducted. Exerting forces and moving objects require the fingers and the hands to be positioned and angled in a way that is appropriate for the performance of the task. The positions of the hands influence the postures of the wrists, elbows, shoulders, and sometimes also the posture of the back and other body parts.

The model has been applied for analyses of grinding, punch press work and fork lift truck driving in industry. In addition, the different work situations were evaluated with methods for analysis of biomechanical loads, spinal shrinkage, postures, and subjective responses (Eklund 1986). From the task analysis, it was judged that the forward force exerted during grinding was the reason for finding that a work chair with a high backrest was advantageous compared to a low backrest. If the task demanded trunk rotation and arm movements to the side due to picking up and handling work pieces, a narrow backrest was found advantageous. The design of punch presses caused restrictions of the knee-room for the operators. A sit-stand seat made it possible to sit closer to the machine and was therefore found advantageous for the back. The movements caused by the handling of work pieces tended to emphasize feelings of insufficient stability on the seat and increased discomfort. Acceleration forces due to velocity changes of the fork lift truck created a demand for increased stability, which was found to be enhanced by increased backrest height and increased seat depth. On the other hand, the task demanded vision to the sides, backwards, and upwards, in order to control the position of the pallets and the traffic. These visual demands were so extensive that substantial movements of the body were required. Trunk movements were found to be facilitated by a low backrest, and restricted by a high one. A 40 cm high backrest was found to be a suitable compromise for driving narrow aisle fork lift trucks.

All these examples demonstrate how the task has a major influence on the choice of optimal design, and also how the design influences the postures, loads and other responses of the workers.

THE CRANE DRIVING TASK

Analyses of crane driving tasks have pointed to certain important task characteristics. In very simple terms, the task can be described as: moving the lift device into position - connecting the goods - lifting - transporting - positioning and lowering the goods - releasing the goods. the crane cabins are often placed 5 - 15 metres above the work level.

In this respect, the task of a crane driver consists of two important factors, namely visual control and operation of the crane. The driver needs a good view of the lifting device and of the goods to be lifted. The visual control is necessary as feedback for the regulation of the lifting device and the goods. Also, control of surrounding factors is needed. The visual angles are consequently mainly determined by two factors. One is the position of the goods, the lifting device, and other areas which need to be overviewed, and the other is the position of the crane driver seat. In the worst case, the goods are placed 15 metres straight below the driver. There may also be visual obstructions, which are of substantial importance. They may originate from objects on the shop floor, from the cabin pillars and the frame of the cabin windows, from the driving seat, from the control panel, from footrests and pedals, and from the driver's own knees and feet. The visual angles necessary for the task and possible for the obstructions will thus determine the head postures and partly also the trunk postures. Furthermore, the lifts and the crane are operated with a number of controls. The design of these will affect the control actions required by the operator and the loadings which arise. Often, the levers used are placed at the front edge of the driver seat. Naturally, the structure and organisation of the task have a strong impact on the temporal pattern of these actions and movements.

Figure 1. Typical work postures for a driver of a conventional crane.

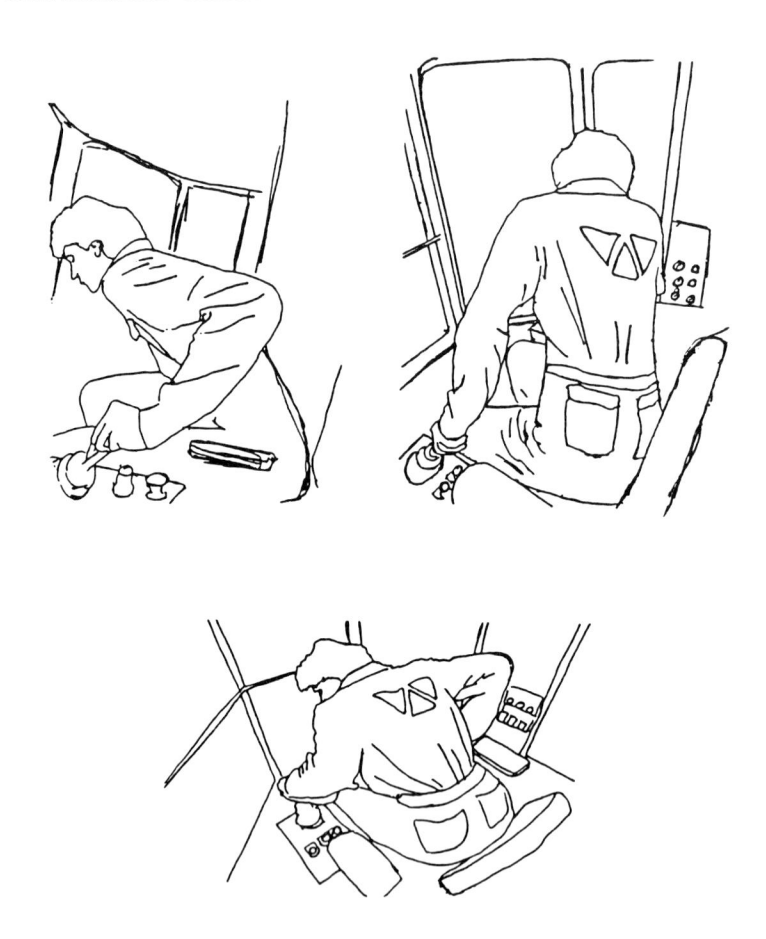

The crane driver's task involves difficult postures during long time periods. An example of three typical postures for drivers of conventional cranes can be seen in Figure 1. In conclusion, analysis of the task and the workplace will show the primary reasons for the work postures chosen.

REFERENCES

Eklund, J., 1986 Industrial seating and spinal loading. Ph.D. Thesis. University of Nottingham.

EVALUATION OF WORK POSTURES
II. Measurement and analysis of work postures in the field

Per Odenrick (+), Jörgen A.E. Eklund (+),
Stefan Zettergren(*), Roland Örtengren (+)

(+) Department of Industrial Ergonomics,
University of Linköping,
S-581 83 Linköping, SWEDEN

(*) Occupational Health Center,
Swedish Steel Corporation (SSAB),
Box 1000, S-613 01 Oxelösund, SWEDEN

INTRODUCTION

Body postures at work can be described by the static position of body segments and the temporal pattern of intersegmental displacements. Both aspects are important in order to make a complete analysis of the musculoskeletal load in a specific work task.

Recording of postures can be performed by direct methods where an electric output signal is generated that is proportional to an intersegmental displacement. Postures can also be recorded by image methods such as video and film. The latter methods give a complete description of posture, but contain much information that is difficult and time-consuming to quantify. Image methods are important as a monitor used simultaneously with the direct methods. A review of current techniques for monitoring motion was presented by Atha (1984).

Two types of direct methods can be used - one where transducers are placed directly on the body and, for example, the angle between two segments is recorded continuously, and the other where markers are placed at specific anatomic points and the displacement of these markers is detected by an optoelectronic equipment or a video scanning system. Body-placed direct recording methods are best suited for measurement of work postures in the field. Two reasons for this are that space at the workplace is often limited and the equipment often is less expensive than an optoelectronic system. The disadvantages are that only one specific dimension is recorded from each transducer and the measurement equipment sometimes imposes an extra load on the subject.

BODY-PLACED DIRECT METHODS

Many transducer principles for body-placed direct recording methods have been used for recording work postures.

Goniometers constructed of levers and electric potentiometers are one common principle. An equipment which measures the head, neck and trunk posture in three dimensions has been developed (Nickometer, SE-ergonomic products, Göteborg, Sweden). The equipment is shown in Figure 1.

Figure 1. An equipment for measurement of head, neck and trunk postures.

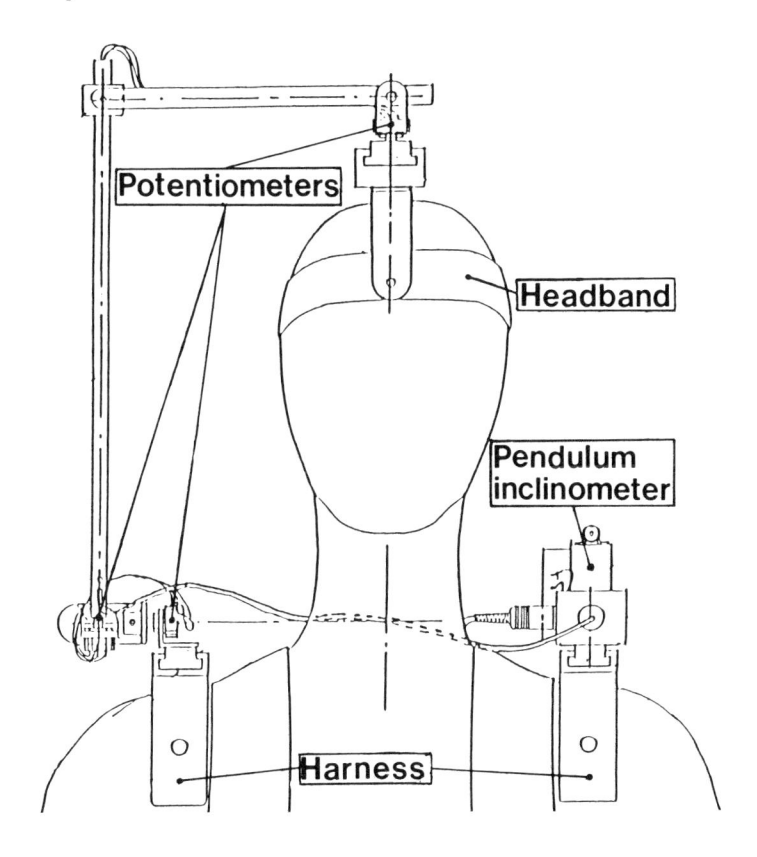

The equipment consist of two main parts, a harness and a headband similar to those used for welding visors. The headband is fastened around the head of the subject. The harness, which consists of a stiff aluminium frame with padding beneath, is placed on the shoulders of the subject and fixed in position with straps around the thorax and elastic braces attached to the waist belt. Its motion is considered to represent the motion of the thorax. Two aluminium rods are connected at a right angle to the harness and the headband. A more detailed description is given below in the present paper.

Elastic strain gauges constructed from thin silicon tubes filled with mercury are used in a system developed at the University of Nottingham (the UNIMAN-system, O'brien 1986). The system consists of a slim suit for the whole body, on which 24 transducers are placed at the major joints and the back. The changes in length of each strain gauge are converted to changes in amplitude of an electric signal by a bridge amplifier. The signal is sampled by a microcomputer system for later processing.

Pendulum inclinometers are often used to measure the position of a body segment, relative to the line of gravity (Nordin et al. 1984). The transducer can be used for measurement of static postures or slow movements. The disadvantage of this transducer is that it is sensitive not only to gravitational acceleration, but also to other acceleration forces and, due to the inertia of the pendulum, overshoot in the signal is often present.

An improved version of the pendulum principle is being developed by Fernandes (1985). The transducer consists of a strain gauge pendulum which decreases errors due to overshoot, although also this transducer is sensitive to acceleration forces.

A new, flexible electrogoniometer was presented by Nicol (1985). The goniometer is sensitive to angular movement and is independent of linear movement in any direction in the plane of motion.

SIGNAL PROCESSING

Signals from the transducers need to be processed prior to the analysis. The type of analysis principally determines the signal processing procedure. For quantification and statistical calculations, it is appropriate to sample the signal, i.e. convert it from analogue to digital form. Before this can be done, the frequency content of the signal must be controlled, so that the time interval between each sample point is short enough to describe every change in the signal level. To present the signal in the frequency domain, the signal must be sampled with a frequency that is at least twice the highest frequency component of the signal. Analogue lowpass filtering is often used for damping the higher frequencies of the signal.

An amplitude histogram corresponding to the probability density function describes the variation of amplitude of a signal. Jointly distributed variables can be described graphically by the bivariate density function and a corresponding two-dimensional histogram can be calculated.

In the analysis of movement signals, it is often necessary to use a static or dynamic biomechanical model to describe the relation between the recorded signals. A static model is adequate in most situations, but if the movements are fast, a dynamic model is necessary to describe the effect of the acceleration forces. Most reported studies on work postures describe moment load, compressive forces etc. by means of a static model, which means that there is a lack of data describing force levels caused by acceleration forces.

AN APPLICATION

The system for measurement of head, neck and trunk posture shown in Figure 1, incorporates three potentiometers placed at the headband and the harness. They are used to record neck flexion-extension in the sagittal plane, lateral head flexion in the frontal plane and head rotation in the transversal plane. A pendulum inclinometer is placed on the harness at the left shoulder to record the inclination of the trunk in the sagittal plane.

The signals from the equipment, and also a sound channel for task identification purposes, are recorded on a seven channel portable tape recorder (TEAC R-71). Reference values for the subject are obtained and recorded by letting the subject stand upright with a straight and balanced head, looking forward and then also performing maximal voluntary flexion, extension, and rotation of the head to the left and to the right. This procedure is performed at the beginning and end of each recording session. For analysis, the tape is played back and the signals are fed into an analysis system built up around a computer (PDP 11/34). The signals are digitized with a sampling rate of 5 Hz per channel. The sampling frequency is determined from the power spectra of the signals. In a study of truck drivers, the maximum frequency for the rotation of the head was found to be 2 Hz.

The signals are also recorded on paper, both for overview monitoring and more detailed visual evaluation of the temporal pattern. A representative portion of 8 minutes from each recording period is chosen for computer analysis.

A purpose-built rig was used in order to perform calibration of the equipment. Calibration measurements are taken with 10 degree increments for all combinations of postures and calibration of the raw signals is performed by the computer. Amplitude histograms are computed and plotted. In addition, a sample from each recording is plotted in an X-Y diagram. This allows a simultaneous description of, for example, head rotation and flexion-extension. In this type of diagram, clusters of points represent common postures taken. The maximal range of voluntary movement for combinations of rotation and flexion-extension can be described in the X-Y plane, as in Figure 2.

Figure 2. An example of maximal voluntary head rotation and flexion-extension of the neck in one subject, described in two dimensions simultaneously.

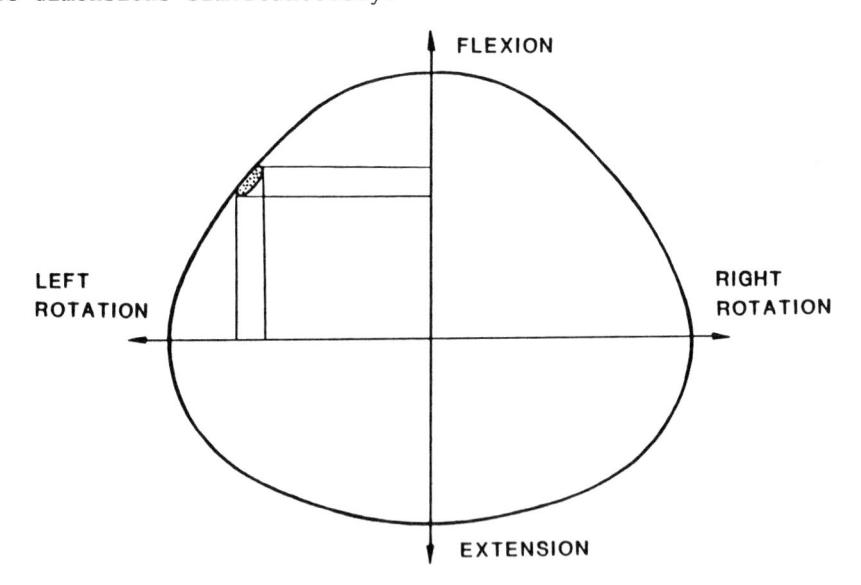

Postures involving combinations of these movements may therefore be substantially closer to the maximum range of motion than indicated by a one-dimensional analysis. The sample of posture shown in Figure 2 is very near the maximal range of voluntary motion, but one-dimensional analyses would indicate the opposite.

DISCUSSION AND CONCLUSIONS

A measurement system for recording postures in the field sets special demands on the equipment compared to a method developed for use in a laboratory. The demands are robust design, battery power supply, easy service of electronic parts, easy transportation between recording sites and resistance to enviromental factors such as ambient temperature, pressure and humidity.

The choice of transducer principle for direct, body-placed recording of posture depends very much on whether a specific part of the body is of interest or if the whole body posture needs to be recorded. The UNIMAN-system is a useful system for whole body recordings, but it does not include head and neck posture. Static inclination of a specific body segment can be recorded by pendulum inclinometers, but the dynamic response of the transducer is limited. The ordinary potentiometer goniometer is sometimes difficult to attach to the body and changes position when fast movements are performed, which leads to poor dynamic characteristics at higher frequencies. The new, flexible goniometer (Nicols 1985) may be a solution that is insensitive to fixation and skin movements.

The signals from the transducer must be processed and analysed on line or stored for later use. For research purposes, it is better to store all data, since other types of analysis may be necessary when information from the first analysis is evaluated. For monitoring purposes, it is better to have a possibility to process data in the field. This can be done if a portable computer is used with software for collecting, processing data and presenting results on a display or a printer.

REFERENCES

Atha J., 1984, Current techniques for measuring motion. Applied Ergonomics, 15.4, 245-257.

Fernandes, A., 1985, Personal communication. Ergonomics Research Unit, University of Surrey.

Nicols, A., 1985, A new flexible electrogoniometer with widespread applications. Proc. 10th International Congress of Biomechanics, Umeå, Sweden. (Arbete och Hälsa 1985:14), p.189.

Nordin M., Örtengren R., Andersson G.B.J., 1984, Measurement of trunk movements during work. Spine, 9, 465-469.

O'Brien, C., 1986, Personal communication. Department of Production Engineering, University of Nottingham.

EVALUATION OF WORK POSTURES
III. Workplace design for crane drivers in a steelworks

Stefan Zettergren (*), Jörgen A.E. Eklund (+),
Per Odenrick (+)

(*) Occupational Health Center,
    Swedish Steel Corporation (SSAB),
    Box 1000, S-613 01 Oxelösund, SWEDEN

(+) Department of Industrial Ergonomics,
    University of Linköping,
    S-581 83 Linköping, SWEDEN

INTRODUCTION
   SSAB, Svenskt Stål AB (Swedish Steel Corporation), Oxelösund, Sweden is an integrated steelworks. The main products are slabs and heavy plate. Production demands a substantial amount of transportation, e.g. raw materials delivered by rail and ship. During successive refinement from one mill to another, several kinds of cranes are involved.
   Crane drivers often complain about discomfort from the neck, shoulders and back, and relate this discomfort to strenuous work postures.
   According to statistics from The National Board of Occupational Safety and Health (Broberg 1984), Swedish crane drivers suffer musculoskeletal injuries and disorders twice as often as expected in a comparison with the average for all other occupations. For female crane drivers, the risk is four to five times higher than that expected for a female working population. Disorders of the neck and shoulders are most frequent, but disorders of the back are also overrepresented.
   In a questionnaire study at Swedish Steel, Borlänge (Sievers 1982), 24% of 58 crane drivers stated that they had been on sick leave in the last 12-month period because of musculoskeletal disorders. A questionnaire study at Swedish Steel, Oxelösund (Runnbeck 1984) showed that among 525 crane drivers, 28% of the male and 70% of the female crane drivers were so affected after 4 to 5 years of employment that they had to consult a doctor and/or a physiotherapist. The most common complaint was aches in the neck and the shoulders, followed by aches in the arms and back. Crane driving is generally considered at the steel plants to be a very

difficult task in this respect, and to have a strong effect on absenteeism.

There are other reports from Sweden with similar results indicating an overrepresentation of musculoskeletal disorders and diseases among crane drivers (Bylund 1978, Lewin 1981), but there are few reports in which the connections between work postures and musculoskeletal strain are described (Thyr 1982, Gustafsson 1984). The task of the crane drivers in this study was to lift and transport steel plates. The crane cabins are placed approximately 10 metres above the ground, and the drivers are seated. The task involves long-distance visual requirements, viewing angles very much below the horizontal and often almost vertical viewing directions downwards and to the sides.

A subjective assessment of the work postures of the crane drivers in a conventional cabin resulted in the following observations: frequent and long duration of flexion in the neck and in the back, frequent and extreme postures of rotation in the neck and the upper thorax, frequent and long duration of abduction and extension in the shoulders, and continuous driving without any opportunities to use the backrest and the armrests while driving. From this assessment, a decision was made that the next design of crane cabin would be movable and turnable in relation to the travelling trolley, and would also have low voltage levels in order to allow smaller levers and operating panels to be incorporated in the armrests, giving less visual obstruction. For comprehensive adjustability, electric motors would be installed. The armrests would then be easily adjustable forward and backward, up and down, and at an angle around a bilateral axis and manually around a vertical axis. It was also decided that the adjustments of the chair up, down and tilting should be driven by electric motors.

The aim of this study was to compare the work postures in a conventional crane design in which the cabin and the lifting devices are constructed as a whole unit, and the postures in a redesigned crane with the cabin separately movable and turnable. The redesigned cabin was also equipped with the improved chair and the new operating lever design described earlier.

EXPERIMENTAL DESIGN

The cranes were chosen so that factors such as types of plate, lift frequencies and work intensity were similar. There were only two drivers, who were well experienced with both cranes. For this reason, only these two female drivers participated in the study. Their ages were 24 and 39 years.

Their heights were 161 and 158 cm respectively. Neither had a history of musculoskeletal disorders.

The measurements took place during the two first hours of the shift. Each driver participated in one morning shift and in one afternoon shift continuously during a period of 40 minutes in each crane. The drivers were instructed to drive in their own normal way in spite of the measurement situation. All measurements were made under ordinary production conditions. Before each measurement session, the neutral position in both standing and sitting was registered and furthermore, the maximum voluntary motion five times in each direction of motion was measured. The recorded motions were the motion of the trunk in the sagittal plane (flexion-extension), the motion of the head in the sagittal plane (flexion-extension), the frontal plane (lateral flexion) and the transversal plane (rotation).

The measurement equipment and method are described in Odenrick, Zettergren, Eklund (1987). Eight representative minutes from each recording were chosen and analysed. On the tape recorder used for recording signals, comments were made on an additional sound channel, e.g. "lifting", "loading", "driving eastward".

RESULTS

The most evident differences were found in trunk flexion and in head rotation. The amplitude histogram in Figure 1 shows trunk flexion for drivers A and B. On the horizontal axis, the angle is described in five-degree intervals and on the vertical axis, relative time in percent of analysed time. In Figure 2, head rotation for driver A and B are presented in a similar way.

Figure 1. Amplitude histograms of the trunk flexion for driver A and B. Solid lines show the redesigned crane and broken lines show the conventional crane.

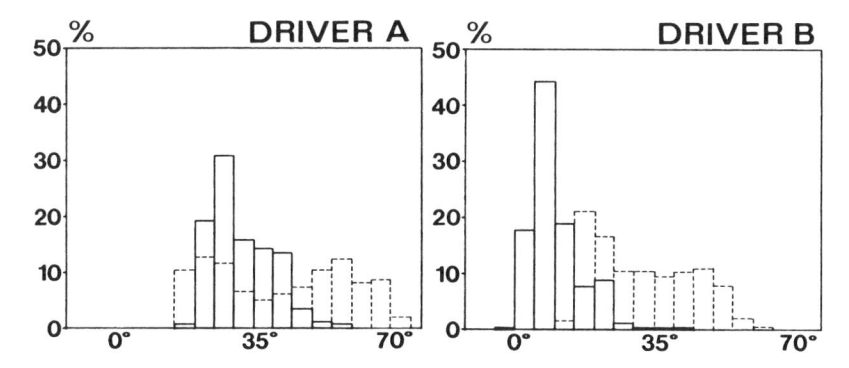

Figure 2. Amplitude histograms of the head rotation for driver A and B. Solid lines show the redesigned crane and broken lines show the conventional crane.

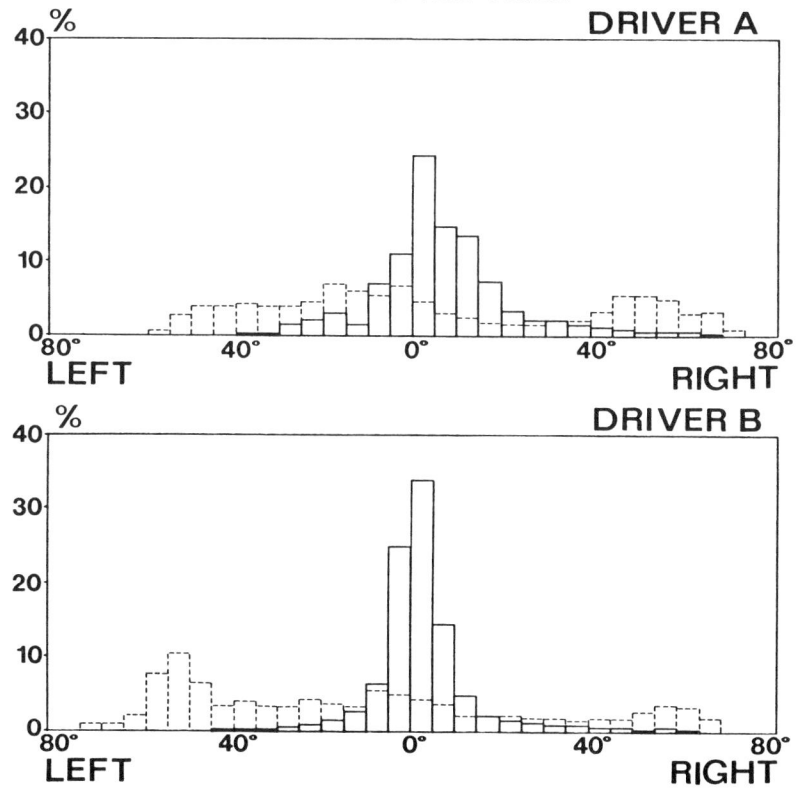

Figure 3. A sample of 400 head postures displayed for driver A in a two-dimensional analysis of flexion-extension and rotation of the head, for the conventional (conv.) and redesigned (redes.) crane.

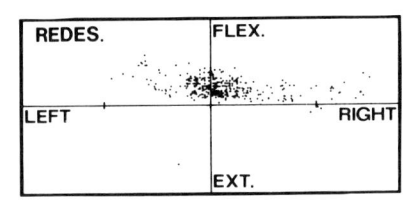

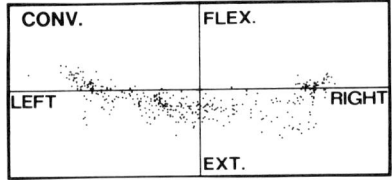

The analyses show a decrease of strenuous postures for the redesigned crane cabin. Trunk flexion 20 degrees or more decreased from 69% to 42% of analysed time, on average. Head flexion-extension was not unambiguously affected. Lateral flexion of the head to the right 5 degrees or more decreased from 20% to 2%, and to the left from 40% to 6% of analysed time, on average. Rotation of the head to the right 15 degrees or more decreased from 31% to 15%, and to the left 15 degrees or more decreased from 43% to 6% of analysed time, on average.

DISCUSSION

The results show clear differences between the two cranes for both the drivers, with clearly decreased time durations in strenuous postures in the redesigned cabin.

As can be seen in the figures, substantial individual differences were present, which requires subjects to be used as their own controls in this type of study.

The results show advantages with the redesigned workplace, regarding the back and neck postures during work, in terms of duration in strenuous postures. The two-dimensional analyses of the temporal pattern in two planes in Figure 3 visualize the differences of the motions of the head. In the same way, the maximal voluntary (or passive) motion in two or three dimensions can be determined in an individual or for a population and then compared with the pattern for a particular workplace.

In the conventional crane, it was common for vision to be demanded in the downward direction. From the measurements, it was noticed that this caused a substantial forward bending of the trunk, but relatively little flexion of the neck.

It was judged that the turnable cabin was the main reason for the decreased head rotation, and the movability of the cabin was the main reason for the decreased forward bending of the trunk. The redesigned control panel and the excluded foot pedals improved vision and were also judged to be of importance for the improved postures. The new chair, the armrests and the new operating levers were perceived as comfortable by the drivers. and they. In spontaneous interviews, the drivers stated that they felt less fatigued after the working day and that they were pleased with the new design.

It is important to determine whether any differences in the distribution of musculoskeletal loading and stress occurs then redesigning complex workplaces such as these. For instance, there may be a different pattern of stress on the hands, wrists and shoulders when working with smaller levers. Factors such as these are important to consider in design evaluations.

REFERENCES

Broberg E., 1984 Belastningsskador i arbetet. National Board of Occupational Safety and Health. Report, ISA 1984:3.

Gustafsson U., 1984 Fast eller ställbar förarstol. Effekter på byggkranförares besvärsupplevelse från rygg- och nack-skulderregion. Report, SAF/LSR, Stockholm.

Odenrick P., Zettergren S., Eklund J.A.E. 1987 Evaluation of work postures II.Measurement and analysis of work postures in the field. Musculoskeletal Disorders at Work, University of Surrey.

Runnbeck L-M., 1984 Traversförarundersökning vid SSAB Oxelösund. Internal report.

Sievers H., 1982 Besvär från rörelseapparaten hos kranförare vid kallvalsverket, SSAB Domnarvet. Report, SAF/LSR, Stockholm.

Thyr L., 1982 Ergonomisk studie av nacken vid en traversarbetsplats. Report, Arbetarskyddsstyrelsen, Umeå.

ONE YEAR'S NOTIFICATIONS OF BACK INJURIES TO THE NATIONAL SOCIAL SECURITY OFFICE, ESPECIALLY WITH RESPECT TO NATURE OF CAUSE, MEDICAL DIAGNOSES AND CONSEQUENCES

K. Josefsen, A.H. Boss, V. Andersen and F. Biering-Sørensen

Laboratory for Back Research, Department TTA & TH, Rigshospitalet, Blegdamsvej 9, DK-2100 Copenhagen Ø, Denmark

---

Summary:
From one year's reports of occupational injuries affecting the back to the National Social Security Office, data describing the causes of injury, the medical diagnoses and the consequences are presented.

The most common causes were object handling, person care and falls. High energy traumas were more often seen to affect men than women. The medical diagnoses were depending on the cause: high energy traumas more commonly gave rise to fractures and contusions. In some groups, when a sudden event had happened during the accident a higher fraction of the injured persons had herniated discs. The consequence of the reported injuries was a large number of lost working days: 93 years of lost working days were found among the 1094 reported cases, but this number is severely underestimated.

In Denmark any occupational injuries to employees must be reported to the National Social Security Office (NSSO). There is made a distinction between occupational accidents (OA) and occupational diseases (OD), according to the duration of the noxious influence from the work. While OAs might be approved independently of the damaged part of the body, the ODs can only be approved for certain diagnoses, known to arise from special working environments. An example of this would be hearing loss among workers exposed to noise.

Physically demanding weight work are however not yet accepted as a cause of back diseases. In order to supplement the documentation describing the problem, all occupational injuries affecting the back and reported to the NSSO in 1978 were examined and analyzed. This article specifically deals with the nature of the causes, diagnoses and consequences.

Materials and methods
As described in a previous article (Andersen V et al, 1987), 39 of 1133 reported cases were excluded for different reasons. Of the 1094 remaining cases, 89% were OAs and 11% were ODs.

Results
Causes. The causes of injury is shown in table 1.

Table 1.
The causes of injury grouped according to occupational accidents and occupational diseases for men and women respectively.

	Occupational Accidents			Occupational Diseases		
	N	Men N=647 %	Women N=330 %	N	Men N=70 %	Women N=47 %
Fall	235	30	12	–	–	–
Stroke, Squeezed	86	12	2	–	–	–
Road Accidents	14	2	1	–	–	–
Person care	248	7	61	19	4	34
Object handling	330	41	20	45	56	13
Bad movement/ posture	46	5	4	27 15	24 4	21 26
Other	16	2	1	2	3	–
Unknown	2	--	–	9	9	6
Total	977	100%	100%	117	100%	100%

Differences were seen among the causes affecting men compared to those affecting women. Thus, all groups of high energy traumas as well as object handling were more common among men than women. Causes affecting women were much dominated by person care because of a large number of nurses and assistant nurses among the women. The differences were also seen among the persons not working as nurses / assistant nurses, however.

Diagnoses
The medical diagnoses, which were made at the time of treatment in hospital or at general practitioner are listed in table 2.

Table 2. Medical diagnoses arising from the injuries, grouped by OAs and ODs as well as by men and women.

	Occupational Accidents			Occupational Diseases		
	N	Men N=647 %	Women N=330 %	N	Men N=70 %	Women N=47 %
Fracture(s)	149	20	6	0	0	0
Contusion	83	10	5	0	0	0
Herniated disc, disc degeneration discopathia sciatica	255	24	30	39	41	21
Spondylosis osteochondrosis spondylolistesis arcolysis Mb. Scheuermann scoliosis	31	4	2	22	21	15
Facet syndrome subluxation, myosis lumbago, distorsion	423	38	53	53	34	62
Osteoporosis, halisteresis	1	0	0	0	0	0
Other	9	1	1	3	3	2
Unknown	26	2	4	0	0	0
	977	100%	100%	117	100%	100%

For both OAs and ODs the most numerous diagnoses belonged to the group of facet syndrome, subluxation, myosis, lumbago and distorsion, while the group of herniated disc, disc degeneration, discopathia and sciatica was also important. Among men fractures and contusions were more common than among women. The opposite was true for the group of facet syndrome, subluxation, myosis, lumbago and distorsion.

The relation between the causes of injury and the diagnoses are listed in table 3.

Table 3.
The diagnoses arising from different causes of injury are listed as percentages of the total number of cases with a reported cause.

	Stroke Squeezed	Fall	Road accident	Object handling	Person care	Bad movement	Other	Not known
Fracture(s)	42	37	43	2	3		13	
Contusion	9	18	7	32	32	28	31	50
Herniated disc disc degeneration discopathia sciatica	24	20	29	1	1	4	6	-
Spondylosis osteochondrosis spondylolistesis arcolysis Mb.Scheuermann scoliosis	-	5	-	2	4	2	6	-
Facet syndrome subluxation, myosis, lumbago, Distorsion	19	17	21	58	56	61	38	-
Osteoporosis, halisteresis	-	1	-	-	-	-	-	-
Other	1	2		1	1	-	6	-
Unknown	5	1		3	5	4	0	50
Total	100%	100%	etc. ...					

High energy traumas most commonly caused fractures. For the object handling group a higher fraction of herniated discs was observed when a sudden event had happened as seen in table 4. This was only the case for the object handling group however. Likewise, none of the other groups of diagnoses showed any major shifts in the two situations.

Table 4. The distribution of diagnoses among OAs in relation to whether a sudden event had happened during person care and object handling.

	Person care		Object handling	
	+ sudden event %	− sudden event %	+ sudden event %	− sudden event %
Herniated disc disc degeneration discopathia sciatica	35	28	53 ←	29
Facet syndrome subluxation, myosis, lumbago, distorsion	48	52	35	58
Others	17	20	12	13
Total	100	100	100	100

Certain occupations were identified in a previous article (Andersen A et al, 1987) as having high notification frequencies. When analyzed in groups of industries however, no major differences between the noxious influence were found. The most numerous causes were: falls, object handling and person care.

Among notifications with fall as cause it was twice as common to fall to another level than on the same level. Within service it was equally common to fall at the same as to another level.

Whether the injured person worked alone at the time of injury was known in about half the cases for the object handling group. In the known cases it was much more common that the injured person worked alone (90%) than with somebody else (10%).

In the person care group, this information was only available in about one third of the cases. Among the known cases 60% had been working alone, 40% had been working with somebody else.

The consequences of the back injuries were evaluated from the number of days the injured person stayed home from work. In 50 percent of the cases this information was available. Among the cases with known period of absence the total number of lost working days was 27.679 (approximately 93 years). As an overall consideration, among OAs the average number of days away from work per injured person were 57 (men: 61, women 49), among the ODs 84 (men 86, women 82). With respect to diagnoses the average number of days away from work per injured person were as follows for OAs: disc diseases 90 days, fractures 83 days, contusions 68 days (diagnosis causing the longest absence periods mentioned) and for ODs: disc diseases 144 days, fractures 65 days (no contusions).

Discussion

The present work clearly states that only a minor part of the injuries were caused by exogenous traumas such as strokes or road accidents. Most of the cases thus arose from noxious influences of short duration occurring during usual work. This is also supported by the fact that "an unusual event" was reported in only very few cases. In another investigation F. Biering-Sørensen (1985), based on reports to the Labour Inspection Service in 1979 found the same: falls were reported as cause in 36% and overstraining in 54% of the cases.

In a previous paper (Andersen V et all, 1987) it was shown that the frequencies of notification were equal for men and women. The causes reported by men were however more often of high energy nature than among women as well as the medical diagnoses were more often fractures and contusions. A tendency to longer periods away from work for men than for women was seen but also longer periods for persons reporting an OD than an OA.

The total number of lost working days is likely to be severely underestimated, since as mentioned information is available from only 50% of the cases. Furthermore among the cases with known period of absence 30 % of the persons were known still to be away from work when the case was reported to the NSSO. Temptations to estimate the total number of lost working days must also take into account that only a fraction of occurred injuries are reported to the NSSO.

To avoid human suffering and reduce the considerable number of working days that are lost because of back injuries, measures might be directed towards the three important causes found in this investigation: falls, object handling and person care. Falls can to a certain extent be prevented with safer working environments. Injuries occurring during object handling and person care must be prevented with better lifting and working instructions and devices for reducing the manipulated loads as well as improved possibilities of taking advantage of these measures in the daily work.

Literature

Andersen, V, Boss, A H, Josefsen, K, Biering-Sørensen, F. One year's notification of back injuries to the National Social Security Office. A demographic description.
(See this volume pages 82-88)

Biering-Sørensen F. Risk of back trouble in individual occupations in Denmark. Ergonomics,1985,28,1;51-60.

AN EPIDEMIOLOGIC STUDY OF POSTURAL RISK FACTORS FOR BACK DISORDERS IN INDUSTRY

L. Punnett, L.J. Fine, W.M. Keyserling

Center for Ergonomics
1205 Beal Avenue
University of Michigan
Ann Arbor, MI   43109   USA

ABSTRACT

A prospective case-referent study of back disorders was conducted in an automobile assembly plant. The objective of this study was to determine if non-neutral trunk postures are risk factors for musculoskeletal disorders of the back. The cases consisted of all workers from the four largest departments in the plant who reported to the medical area with back pain over a ten month period. The referents were randomly selected from all workers in the same departments who did not report to the medical area for back or shoulder pain during this period. One hudred and eighteen cases and 259 referents were interviewed and examined. Each case was examined on average 49 days (median 28 days) after selection. In addition, each worker's job was filmed and analyzed in order to characterize the postural and peak force requirements on the low back.

Eighty-three per cent of all the workers were required to work at least briefly during each job cycle in trunk flexion greater than 45 degrees, and 45% in a trunk twist or lateral bend posture. All three of these postures were significant predictors of low back disorders among cases with positive findings on interview (odds ratios 4.9, 5.7 and 5.9 respectively). The odds ratio for low back disorders among workers who used both mild and severe flexion was 5.1 ($p = 0.02$); among those who used both mild flexion and twisting it was 7.3 ($p = 0.003$). Peak low back forces were relatively low among all subjects (mean 482lb, median 447lb) and did not appear to be confounding variables for the above measures of association. These results may be of assistance in the design of workstation layout and job requirements.

RISK FACTORS AND BACK PAIN

R.W. Porter

Consultant Orthopaedic Surgeon, Doncaster Royal Infirmary, Armthorpe Road, Doncaster, DN2 5LT, UK

Many have suggested that the prevention of low back pain will result from the correct design of the working environment (Snook et al 1978), but with such a vast problem we should also consider the potential of prediction, and attempt to identify subjects at risk.

There is no single test that will identify a potential back pain sufferer, probably because back pain is only a symptom resulting from many different pathologies each of which have a multifactorial aetiology. Some of these factors however have been identified, and as they are more fully understood, it should be possible to make useful predictions.

1 One of the most reliable indicators of future back pain, is a history of pain (Buckle et al 1980, Roland et al 1983 and Drinkall et al 1984). This is particularly significant if absence of 5-6 weeks follow a fall, and if there is persisting disability with restricted straight leg raising, and weakness of hip and abdominal flexors (Troup et al 1981). A man is at poor risk entering a heavy labouring industry with a previous history of back pain, but unfortunately prediction at this stage is too late to influence the back pain problem. For the young recruit, an uneventful past history is an insensitive predictive measure.

2 Our family history studies have confirmed a familial aspect to annular fissure, and disc protrusion. We compared the first degree relatives of fifty discectomy patients with those of fifty matched subjects, and noted that forty six of the 192 first degree relatives of the discectomy patients had 'significant' low back pain, compared with 19 of 155 first degree relatives of the

control subjects ($x = 6.39$, $p < 0.02$). We were not able to identify any difference in the HLA antigens of the two groups. Family history and perhaps genetic and biochemical indices may prove relevant as fundamental research continues (Jayson et al 1984).

3 Anthropometric studies are sometimes conflicting, but there is some evidence that taller men have a disproportionate amount of back pain absenteeism (Lawrence 1955, Hrubec and Nashbold 1975, and Tauber 1970).

Pelvic height may be an important component (Merriam et al 1983).

We observed a greater general practice attendance with back pain in a mining village where the seam was 1.67 cm compared with a second village with a 1.2 m seam (Porter and Hibbert 1986). Men crawl in a lower seam and suffer less stress than from stooping in a higher seam. Weight and body build however, have not been shown to have any consistent association with back pain experience (Hirsch et al 1969, Gyntelberg 1974, Karavonen et al 1980).

4 Isometric strength relative to the demands of the job, are a risk factor for both episodes and severity of back pain absenteeism (Chaffin and Park 1973, Keyserling et al 1980). There is some evidence that fitness and strength protects an individual from the effects of a disc protrusion. Our data comparing the proportion of men attending hospital with criteria of disc protrusion, showed a significantly lower proportion of miners than men from other occupations amongst all back pain clinic attenders ($p < 0.01$). This is more marked when examining men admitted with disc lesions, and very few miners required discectomy (Table 1). It suggests that the heavy manual work of mining protects the annulus from serious failure, or strengthens the posterior longitudinal ligament, resisting the effects of a disc protrusion. Conversely, light work confers a risk of disc protrusion. This agrees with Kelsey's (1975) observation, that disc protrusion is more common amongst sedentary workers.

5 Early work experience confers a relative risk influence in different back pain syndromes. We asked men attending a back pain clinic to complete an occupational questionnaire, to determine whether there was a relationship between heavy lifting in early life, and the relative incidence of four defined back pain syndromes. Men fulfilling criteria for symptomatic disc protrusion, had done significantly less heavy lifting between 15 and

20 years of age, than men with root entrapment syndrome, segmental instability and neurogenic claudication ($\alpha <$ 0.001). Work in early life confers a selective risk, heavy work protecting a man from symptomatic disc protrusion, but increasing his risk of developing syndromes associated with degenerative change.

6 The small vertebral canal is an important factor in several back pain syndromes (Verbiest 1954, Ehni 1969, Porter et al 1980, Rothman and Simone 1982), and is probably the most important of the predictors of back pain. It is only a relative predictor. Many individuals with a small vertebral canal will never have back pain, because they develop no secondary pathology. When a small canal is compromised by disc protrusion, bony or soft tissue degenerative change, or by segmental instability it readily produces compression or ischaemic changes in the cauda equina or roots. A subject with similar pathological changes in a larger canal, may escape symptoms.

We observed that almost half the patients attending hospital with disc symptoms had sagittal measurements of the vertebral canal below the tenth percentile for the general population (Porter et al 1978). When a symptomatic protrusion occurs, the response to treatment is related to canal size (Kornberg and Rechtine 1985).

Patients with back pain attending a general practitioner have smaller canals than matched controls (Drinkall et al 1984). Absenteeism in 50 year old miners is more common in subjects with small canals (MacDonald et al 1984).

The vertebral canal can be measured by ultrasound, which is well suited for screening purposes, being safe, non-invasive and relatively quick to perform (Hibbert et al 1981). The repeatability by this technique has been estimated between 0.3 and 1.0 mm, (Hibbert et al 1981, Legg and Gibbs 1984), compared with a sagittal range of about 11 - 22 mm (Huizinga et al 1951). Ultrasound has not yet been used for screening, but prospective studies continue to assess its importance.

7 Radiological investigation has little value in predicting low back pain. A critical review of radiographs of the spine led the NIOSH and American Conference of Radiologists to conclude that it was 'of little assistance in predicting future trauma or disability from on-the-job stress' (1974). Montgomery (1976) reached the same conclusion reviewing many of the large studies.

The demonstration of isthmic spondylolysis or spondylolisthesis is sometimes viewed as a serious risk factor, but this is not our experience. We observed 131 patients with lysis of the pars interarticularis in 2360 patients attending a first referral hospital back pain clinic (Porter & Hibbert 1984), an incidence no greater than the incidence of defects in the general population (Roche & Rowe 1951). The lysis appears to widen the vertebral canal and protect the patient from cauda equina symptoms. A symptomatic disc protrusion or neurogenic claudication is unusual in a patient with a pars defect. They are more prone to instability symptoms of back pain and referred pain, but the demonstration of a lytic pars defect without symptoms, should not affect a man's employment.

8 The manner in which pain is percieved, and the response it produces is not directly related to the pathology and the pain source. Personality and motivation greatly affects the incidence of back pain. In hospital and general practice surveys, increased anxiety, neurosis, depression and heightened somatic awareness have been found in back pain populations, (Lloyd et al 1979, Crown 1978, Forrest & Wolkind 1974, Frymoyer et al 1985). It would be helpful if such individuals could be identified in early life. The imprinting of abnormal pain behaviour will be present in the early years (Melzak 1973, Letham et al 1983), but it has not yet been identified by a prospective study. One may speculate that a good history a record of school absenteeism and a suitable psychological questionnaire would help.

We are now in a position to predict that a man with a small vertebral canal, a strong family history of relatives with previous disc protrusion, whose work between 15 and 20 years of age did not involve heavy lifting is at considerable risk of developing a symptomatic disc protrusion. Another man with a small vertebral canal engaged in lifting occupations in early life is at risk of developing syndromes of back pain related to degenerative change (root entrapment, instability, and neurogenic claudication). A man at least risk is one with a large vertebral canal, who has no relatives with previous disc symptoms, who develops and maintains a strong spine in early life and avoids acute and chronic spinal injury.

There are some occupations where it is not possible to produce an ideal working environment. Men working in these situations deserve the benefit of pre-employment screening, once we can be confident about combined risk factors.

Buckle PW, Kember PA, Wood AD et al. 1980. Spine: 5; 254-258. Factors influencing occupational back pain in Bedfordshire.

Chaffin DB, Park KS. 1973. American Industrial Hygiene Association 34: 513-525. A longitudinal study of low back pain as associated with occupational weight lifting factors.

Crown S. 1978. Rheumatology and Rehabilitation 17: 114-123. Psychological aspects of low back pain.

Drinkall JN et al. 1984. British Medical Journal. The value of ultrasonic measurement of the spinal canal diameter in general practice. 288:121-122

Ehni G. 1969. Journal of Neurology 31: 490-494. Significance of the small lumbar spinal canal: cauda equina compression syndromes due to spondylolysis.

Forrest AJ, Wolkind SH. 1974. Rheumatology and Rehabilitation 13: 148-153. Masked depression in men with low back pain.

Frymoyer JW et al. 1985. Clinical Orthopaedics 195: 178-184. Psychological factors in low back pain disability.

Gyntelberg F. 1974. Danish Medical Buletien 21: 30-36. One year incidence of low back pain among male residents of Copenhagen aged 40-59.

Hibbert CS et al 1981. British Journal of Radiology 54: 905-907. Measurement of the lumbar spinal canal by diagnostic ultrasound.

Hirsch C et al. 1969. Clinical Orthopaedics 63: 171-176. Low back pain symptoms in a Swedish female population.

Hrubec A and Nashbold. 1975. American Journal of Epidemiology 102: 366-376. Epidemiology of lumbar disc lesions in the military in World War II.

Huizinga J et al 1951. Physical Anthropolometry 30: 22-23. The human lumbar vertebral canal: a biometric study.

Jayson MIV et al. 1984. Lancet 2: 1186-1187. A fibrinolytic defect in chronic back pain syndromes.

Karavonen et al. 1980. Scandanavian Journal of Rehabiliation Medicine 12: 53-60. Back and leg complaints in relation to muscle strength in young men.

Kelsey JL. 1975. Rheumatology and Rehabilitation 14: 144-159. An epidemiological study of acute herniated lumbar intervertebfal discs.

Keyserling et al. 1980. Journal of Occupational Medicine 22: 332-336. Isometric strength testing as a means of controlling medical incidents on strenuous jobs.

Kornberg M and Rechtine GR. 1985. *Spine* 10: 328-330. Quantitative assessment of the fifth lumbar spinal canal by computed tomography in symptomatic L4-L5 disc disease.

Lawrence JS. 1955. *British Journal of Industrial Medicine* 12: 249-261. Rheumatism in coal miners: occupational factors.

Legg SJ and Gibbs V. 1984. *Spine* 9: 79-82. Measurement of the lumbar spinal canal by echo ultrasound.

Letham J at al 1983. *Behaviour Research Therapy* 21: 401-408. Outline of a fear avoidance model of exaggerated pain perception.

Lloyd et al. 1979. *Rheumatology and Rehabilitation* 18: 30-34. A psychiatric study of patients with persistent low back pain.

Macdonald et al. 1984. *Journal of Occupational Medicine* 26: 23-28. The relationship between spinal canal diameter and back pain in coal miners: ultrasonic measurement a screening test?

Melzack R. 1973. *The Puzzle of Pain*. Penguin Books Ltd, Harmondsworth, Middlesex, England.

Merriam WF et al. 1983. *Journal of Bone and Joint Surgery*. 65-B: 153-156. A study revealing a tall pelvis in subjects with low back pain.

Montgomery CH. 1976. *Journal of Occupational Medicine* 18: 495-498. Pre-employment back x-rays.

Porter R W and Hibbert CS. 1984. *Spine* 9: 755-758. Symptoms associated with lysis of the pars interarticularis.

Porter R W and Hibbert CS. 1986. *Clinical Biomechanics* 1: 7-10. Back pain and neck pain in four general practices.

Porter R W et al 1980. *Spine* 8: 99-105. Backache and the lumbar spinal canal.

Porter R W et al 1978. *Journal of Bone and Joint Surgery* 60-B: 485-487. The size of the lumbar spinal canal in the symptomatology of disc lesions.

Present AJ. 1974. *Radiology* 112: 229-230. Radiography of the lower back in pre-employment physical examinations. ACR-NIOSH Conference.

Roche MB and Rowe GG. 1951. *Anat Rec* 109: 233-252. The incidence of separated neural arch and coincident bone variations: a survey of 4200 skeletons.

Roland et al. 1983. *British Medical Journal* 286: 523-525. Can general practitioners predict the outcome of episodes of back pain?

Rothman RH and Simone FA. 1982. The Spine. Second Edition
W B Saunders Company, Philadelphia, London, Toronto.
p 518.

Snook SH et al. 1978. Journal of Occupational Medicine
20: 478-481. A study of three preventative approaches
to low back injury.

Tauber J. 1970. Journal of Occupational Medicine. 12:
128-130. An orthodox look at backaches.

Troup JDG et al. 1981. Spine 6: 61-69. Back pain in
industry. A prospective survey.

Verbiest H. 1954. Journal of Bone and Joint Surgery.
36-B: 230-237. A radicular syndrome from developmental
narrowing of the lumbar vertebral canal.

Table 1. Back pain in male adults and miners in a hospital catchment area over 3 years.

Sample	Number	% Miners
Time averaged mean of the adult, male population, employed and in the hospital catchment area	~80 000	~21
Male back pain clinic attenders	1 422	31
Men with criterion of disc protrusion	250	20
Men admitted with symptoms of disc protrusion	70	14
Men undergoing surgery for disc protrusion	33	9

ONE YEAR'S NOTIFICATIONS OF BACK INJURIES TO THE NATIONAL SOCIAL SECURITY OFFICE. A DEMOGRAPHIC DESCRIPTION

V. Andersen, A.H. Boss, K. Josefsen and F. Biering-Sørensen

Laboratory for Back Research, Department TTA & TH, Rigshospitalet, Blegdamsvej 9, DK-2100 Copenhagen Ø, Denmark

Summary
Back trouble is a frequent reason for work absence and cause of considerable expenses for the national health in Denmark. In Denmark any employee must be insured against occupational injuries. Although there is a significant underreporting of notifications of occupational injuries it is considered that the most serious injuries are reported. The investigation includes one year of notifications of occupational back injuries to NSSO. This article describes the IP with regard to gender, age, civil status, distribution on industry and occupation, seniority, salary pay conditions, geographical place of work, hour, day and month of accident, the time elapsed from the accident until the notification as well as the decision regarding compensation taken by NSSO.

Background
Back trouble is a frequent reason for work absence and cause of considerable expenses for the national health in Denmark (Pedersen,1980,Biering-Sørensen,1983).Many cases of back trouble are considered to be of occupational origin. In Denmark any employee must be insured against occupational injuries (Industrial Injuries Act,1978). Employers,doctors and dentists must report occupational Injuries, and the injured person (IP) or his trade union may report. Notification may be given either to the Labour Inspection Service (Arbejdstilsynet) (LIS) or to The National Social Security Office, Industrial Injuries Insurance (Sikringsstyrelsen, Arbejdsskadeforsikringen) (NSSO). The purpose of notification to LIS is to prevent accidents, while NSSO deal with questions regarding compensation.
Although there is a significant underreporting of notifications of occupational injuries it is considered that the most serious injuries are reported for the purpose of compensation. It was therefore of interest to investigate the notifications of back injuries that had reached NSSO.
The investigation includes one year of notifications of occupational back injuries to NSSO. This article describes the IP with regard to gender, age, civil status, distribution on industry and occupation, seniority, salary pay conditions, distribution of workplace on geography, hour, day and month of accident, the time elapsed from the accident until the notification as well as the decision regarding compensation taken by NSSO.
The purpose of the present investigation is to identify risk-populations among persons with occupational back injuries.

Law
In Denmark any employee (paid or unpaid) must be insured against occupational injuries (Industrial Injuries Act). The employer must report occupational injuries to his insurance company and doctors and dentists to NSSO. Section 9 in this law states occupational injuries as:
1. Accidents caused by the work or the circumstances of the work.
2. Injurious effects of not more than a few days duration. This is legally considered as accidents.
3. Occupational diseases according to a list, but as no back disease are listed each case had to be specifically proved.

The Industrial Injuries Act which form the basis of NSSO had been valid from 1st. April 1978, before which another law was used (Insurance Against the Effects of Occupational Accidents). The difference between the two laws mainly concerns the treatment of the compensations.
A special act (Drafted Personal Injuries Act) applies to drafted personal in military service.

Delimitation
Due to difficulties in using NSSO' method to distinguish between occupational accidents and occupational diseases a more simple one was used in this investigation.
Occupational accidents (OA) are here delimitated as occurring from one specific event, usually momentary or of no more than one day's duration, and occupational diseases (OD) as occurring during a period, i.e. more than one day. The classification by NSSO of accidents and diseases was deduced from the registration numbers of the case records in NSSO .

Materials and methods
1133 notifications regarding back and spine reached NSSO in 1978.
The information comes from the notification formula, medical certificates and corresponds between NSSO and the IP.
The following information was recorded:
Personal: year of birth, gender and civil status.
Occupational: industrial and occupational code, postal area coding for the workplace, salary pay conditions and seniority.
Nature of injury: OA or OD. For OA time, day and month of accident. The event in relation to the accident.
Date of notification.
Medical diagnosis: diagnosis by specialist if existing, otherwise the first consulted doctor.
Number of days away from work due to the present back injury.
Decision taken by NSSO : decision, possible social and medical disability.
Statistics. Poisson distribution with 95% confidence limit was used with the exception of time of accident, time elapsed from accident to notification and approved versus rejected cases, where chi square test was used.

Results

39 cases were excluded, most of which were drafted personal performing military service. The investigation was therefore based on 1094 cases. 89% (977) were OA and 11% (117) were OD according to the delimitation given above. In 17 cases this was in disagreement with the division made by NSSO .
Gender. Among OA 66% (647) were men and 34% (330) women and among OD 60% (70) men and 40% (47) women. This was the same distribution as in the total Danish working population (National Bureau of Statistics,1979,1).
Age. The frequency of notification of OA was highest for persons between 25-30 and 49 years of age. For OD a tendency for higher frequencies of notification among the younger was seen (less than 40 years of age) than among the older persons (National Bureau of Statistics,1979,2).
Civil status. No differences were found between the civil status of the IP and the total Danish working population (National Bureau of Statistics,1979,2).
Industry. The distribution on industry was: 43% (39-47%) within services, 22% (18-24%) within manufacturing, 11% (9-13%) within transport,storage and communication and 17% (15-20%) on the remaining occupations while 8% (6-9%) were unknown.
In Table 1 the notification frequencies of the back injuries are classified according to the International Standard Industrial Classification of all economic activities (ISIC) from 1968. Only transport,storage and communication had a significant higher frequency of notification than the remaining major groups in ISIC. High frequencies were found within bus service as well as within slaughtering, schools, hospitals and welfare institutions
Among the 206 IP within hospitals and sanatoriums 94 were assistent nurses,41 nurses, 31 hospitals porters and 4 medical doctors. Among the 153 within welfare institutions 71 were assistant nurses, 11 nurses, 6 hospitals porters and 4 pedagogues.
Occupation. The frequencies of notifications is shown for major occupational groups and subgroups with more than 5 notifications in Table 2. No information exist for total Denmark on the numbers of persons in individual occupations for 1978, why notification frequencies were calculated on the basis of information regarding 1980 (National Bureau of Statistics,1981).
There was no differences in notification frequencies for women engaged as salaried employers, skilled or unskilled workers.For men, however, the frequencies increased along the mentioned groups and especially male unskilled workers had significant higher notification frequencies than the average.
The exceptional high frequency of notification for the group of doormen, liftmen etc. is probably due to discrepancies in the demarcation of the occupations in this investigation and the reference used.
High frequencies were found among farmers assistants, woodmen and fisher assistants as well as slaughters, building workers and military officers and again nurse assistants and nurses.

Frequencies of notifications calculated on the basis of information from the trade-unions were (for each 1000 in work) 2.4 (1.8-3.2) for nurses, 8.8 (7.2-9.9) for nurse assistants and 9.8 (6.8-13.5) for hospital porters.
Seniority. 25% of the persons who had notified an OA had a seniority of 12 months or less. Significant more men (22%) than women (13%) with an notified OA had a seniority of more than 8 year's. This differences didn't show up for OD. For 16-20 % the seniority were unknown.
Salary pay condition. No difference was found between the pay conditions for IP notifying OA or OD. For those occupational groups which belongs under the Danish Employers' Association there was a lower frequency of piece-workers than in the comparable groups in the present study. For 12% the salary pay condition were unknown.
Geographical distribution of the workplace. No differences were found between persons living in the bigger cities or in the rural areas.
The time of the accidents. The accidents happened, not unexpected, in the daytime with maximae from 10 a.m. to noon and from 2 to 4 p.m. Significant more accidents happened on Mondays than on other working days and during august to November (incl.) than during the other 4-months periods of the year.
Elapsed time from accident to notification. 25 % of the accidents were reported within a week, 50 % within 2 weeks and 95 % within 8 months.
Decisions of approved versus rejected cases taken by NSSO is shown in Table 3. OA were more frequent approved than OD, likewise men had higher approval rates than women.

Discussion
In Denmark as well as in other countries occupational injuries are underreported (Biering-Sørensen,1985). This may vary for different occupational groups, types of accidents etc. It is therefore apparent that the 1133 cases in this investigation only describes a fraction of all actual back injuries in 1978. It is to be expected however, that for the purpose of compensations the reported cases represent the most serious ones.
The higher frequency of notification of OD among younger than elderly may be due to a particular underreporting of OD among elderly. They may more easily accept attrition as a part of the work than the younger while the most serious or obvious OA are always reported. Selection out of an occupation or promotion to supervision jobs etc. may contribute.
The more frequent notification by nurses, nurse assistants, hospital porters, fisher workers and slaughter workers are confirmed by earlier investigations (Vanggård & Nielsen,1977, Biering-Sørensen,1981, Kristensen,1985).
It was not possible to obtain data concerning the seniority for the total Danish occupational population. It can be expected that OD develops over a span of years and therefore, that the IP who notify an OD had a higher seniority than persons who notify an OA. This was partially confirmed since the group with a low seniority made up a greater part of the OA than the OD. It must be taken into account, however, that the investigation registered the seniority at the latest job only. In addition attitudes towards reporting might influence the obtained results.

Musculoskeletal disorders at work

Table 1. Distribution on industry of persons with a reported back injury to the Danish National Social Security Office in 1978. Only the most numerous (>10) subgroups are listed. Notification frequencies are calculated per 1000 persons in the occupation. (95% confidens interval in brackets).

	number of notifications N=1094	frequency of notification based on ref from 1976		frequency of notification based on ref from 1978	
AGRICULTURE, FORESTRY AND FISHING	52	0.3	(0.2-0.3)	0.3	(0.2-0.4)
agriculture specified	25	0.1	(0.1-0.2)	0.2	(0.1-0.3)
other agriculture	11	1.0	(0.5-1.9)		
fishing	12	1.0	(0.6-1.9)	1.0	(0.5-1.7)
MANUFACTURING	235	0.5	(0.4-0.5)	0.4	(0.4-0.5)
slaughterhouses	31	1.4	(1.0-2.0)		
timber industry	11	0.8	(0.4-1.5)		
chemical raw mat. industry	10	0.8	(0.4-1.5)		
engine production	28	0.4	(0.3-0.6)		
electroindustry	17	0.5	(0.3-0.8)		
shipbuilding yard	17	0.6	(0.4-0.6)		
CONSTRUCTION TOTAL	81	0.4	(0.3-0.5)	0.4	(0.3-0.5)
contractor service	22	0.4	(0.2-0.6)		
bricklayer firms	13	0.4	(0.2-0.6)		
carpenter business	20	0.5	(0.3-0.8)		
COMMERCE	39	0.1	(0.1-0.1)	0.1	(0.1-0.2)
TRANSPORT, STORAGE & COMMUNICATION	121	0.7	(0.6-0.9)	0.7	(0.6-0.9)
railroad	26	1.1	(0.7-1.6)		
busservice	10	4.4	(2.2-7.9)		
carrying van trade	17	0.5	(0.3-0.8)		
sea-borne carriage	28	1.0	(0.7-1.4)		
post, telecommunication	15	0.3	(0.2-0.6)		
BANKING & INSURANCE	9	0.1	(0.0-0.1)	0.1	(0.0-0.1)
SERVICE TOTAL	471	0.4	(0.3-0.4)	0.6	(0.6-0.7)
police & court	11				
defence	30				
education	10				
hospital, sanatorium	206			0.9	(0.8-1.0)
welfare institutions	153				
TOTAL INDUSTRIES	1094	0.4	(0.4-0.5)	0.4	(0.4-0.5)
UNKNOWN	86	1.1	(0.9-1.3)	3.9	(3.2-4.9)

Table 2. Distribution on occupation of persons with a reported back injury to the Danish National Social Security Office in 1978. Only the most numerous subgroups (>5) are listed. Notification frequencies are calculated per 1000 persons in the occupation. (95% confidence interval in brackets).

	MEN			WOMEN		
	Total number N=717	Frequency per 1000		Total number N=377	Frequency per 1000	
SELF EMPLOYED	11	0.04	(0.0-0.1)	0		
HELPMATE	0			1	0.01	(0.0-0.1)
EMPLOYEE & CIVIL SERVANT	129	0.2	(0.2-0.3)	246	0.4	(0.4-0.5)
officer in military	17	2.2	(1.3-3.6)	0		
nurse	5	2.6	(1.1-6.3)	48	1.0	(0.7-1.3)
assistant nurse	11	0.9	(0.4-1.7)	155	2.1	(1.7-2.4)
policeman	6	0.3	(0.1-0.7)	0		
clerk	5	0.1	(0.1-0.3)	6		
superior in shop	16			0		
shop assistant	2	0.1	(0.0-0.2)	8	0.1	(0.1-0.3)
foreman	11			0		
SKILLED WORKER	203	0.7	(0.6-0.8)	9	0.5	(0.3-0.9)
slaughter	16	1.0	(0.6-1.6)	2		
printer	6			0		
smith	20			0		
machine worker	21	0.7	(0.5-1.0)	0		
mechanic	7			0		
motor mechanic	9	0.8	(0.5-1.0)	9		
machine fitter	18			0		
brick layer	9			1		
carpenter	34	0.9	(0.8-1.4)	0		
house carpenter	7			0		
electrician	5	0.1	(0.1-0.3)	0		
apprentice unspecified	6			0		
UNSKILLED	360	1.1	(1.0-1.3)	119	0.4	(0.3-0.4)
agriculture assistant	15			0		
forestry assistant	8	2.1	(1.1-2.3)	0		
fisher assistant	9			0		
navvy	8			0		
sailor	13			0		
driver	51	0.8	(0.6-1.1)	2		
harbor policeman	5			0		
store & storehouse worker	7			0		
hospitalporter	37			0		
porter,elevatorman etc.	29	16	(10-23)	2		
cleaning,kitchen etc.	4			42		
homehelper,daynurse	2	0.6	(0.2-1.3)	31	0.3	(0.3-0.4)
factory worker	132			31		
UNKNOWN	14	0.2	(0.1-0.4)	2	0.02	(0-0.1)
TOTAL OCCUPATIONS	717	0.48	(0.44-0.51)	377	0.33	(0.29-0.36)

Table 3.
The decision of approved versus rejected cases taken by the Danish National Social Security Office for occupation acccidents (OA) and occupational diseases (OD).

	Men		Women	
	OA N=647	OD N=70	OA N=330	OD N=47
approved	58%	7%	39%	4%
rejected	30%	87%	47%	91%
shelved case	12%	6%	15%	4%

Concerning time of accidents, studies on hospitals has shown high incidences in the morning, in the late afternoon and at bedtime. The higher number of notifications in the autumn couldn't be explained sufficiently by more working days nor by accession of young inexperienced people just finished school, although the latter might contribute.
A considerably delay of the notification of OA was found. According to Danish law OA must be reported within 8 days, but this was done in only 1/4 of the cases.
Very few OD were approved compare to the OA. This was to be expected as back diseases were not listed as occupational diseases in reference to Danish law and thus had to be justified in each case.
The frequency of approved cases was higher for men than for women. This is in accordance with the higher frequencies of high-energy traumas for men as is shown in a following article (Josefsen et al,1987).

References
Biering_Sørensen,F. A prospective study of low back pain in a general population. III Medical service - work consequence. Scand.J.Rehab.Med, 1983,15,89-96.
Biering-Sørensen,F.,Vejerslev,L.O.,Gyntelberg,F. Anmeldte rygskader ved håndtering blandt hospitalsansatte.Ugeskr.læg. 1981,15,947-51.
Biering-Sørensen,F. National statistics in Denmark - back trouble versus occupation. Ergonomics,1985,28,1;25-29.
Drafted Personal Injuries Act, Lov om erstatning til skadelidte værnepligtige m.fl. Lov nr.80 af 8.marts 1978.
Industrial Injuries Act, Lov om arbejdsskadeforsikring. Lov nr.79 af 8.marts 1978.
Insurance Against the Effects of Occupationa Accidents, Ulykkesforsikringsloven. Lov om forsikring mod følger af ulykkestilfælde. Lovbekendtgørelse nr.137 af 26.4.1968, med ændringer.
Josefsen,K., Boss,A.H., Andersen,V., Biering-Sørensen,F. One year's notifications of back injuries to the National Social Security Office, especially with respect to nature of cause, medical diagnosis, and consequences. See this volume.
Kristensen,T.S. The occupational environment and health of slaughterhouse workers V. Low back pain and absense of acount of low back syndromes. Ugeskr.læg 1985;147:3276-83.
National Bureau of Statistics (1), Danmarks statistik. Registerfolketællingen. Kommuner. Statistisk tabelværk 1979;1,bind 2.
National Bureau of Statistics, Danmarks statistik. Folke- og boligtællingen 1. Jan 1980. L 1 Landstabelværk. Danmarks statistik, 1981.
National Bureau of Statistics (2), Danmarks statistik. Statistiske efterretninger. Arbejdsstyrkeundersøgelsen. Danmarks statistik, 1979.
United Nations: ISIC: International Standard Industrial Classification, statistical papers 1968; Senes,M, No.4, Rev.2, add.1.
Vanggård,L.,Nielsen,S. Arbejdsmiljøet i dansk fiskeri. Ugeskr.læg.1977,7,413-419.

WORKING POSTURES AND SPINAL DISEASES AMONG PORPHYRY QUARRYMEN

D. Colombini[x], E. Occhipinti[x], A. Cristofolini[xx], A. Grieco[x]

[x] "Ergonomics of Posture and Movement" Research Unit (E.P.M.) - Via S.Barnaba, 8 - Milan (Italy)

[xx] Occupational Health Service, Trento (Italy)

INTRODUCTION

Over 100 porphyry quarries, employing about 1400 workers, are concentrated in a small valley in Northern Italy.

The working postures of the quarrymen were analysed and evaluated and parallelly the occurrence of cervical, thoracic and lumbosacral diseases among 1157 quarrymen were studied by means of a suitably designed questionnaire.

The clinical results obtained in three different groups of quarrymen, each stratified into four age sub-groups, were compared with those obtained in paired control groups consisting of age- and sex-matched subjects who had never been exposed to occupational hazards for the spine.

The aim of the study was to ascertain whether in fact postural and mechanical stresses play an effective role in the etiopathogenesis of spinal diseases in quarrymen.

METHODS

The main jobs common to all porphyry quarries were studied: a) caterpillar driver (operating a vehicle for the movement of rough stone and pallets of finished products); b) sorter (sorting and manual loading of porphyry slabs weighing from 10 to 35 Kg on special pallets); stone cutter (cutting stones into required sizes using a power hammer) (Fig. 1).

The study of the work postures and manual handling in these three groups of workers was carried out mainly using biomechanical methods developed by the authors (Colombini. et al.,1985). In particular, stresses on lumbar disks during the various phases of work were measured. In parallel, the cardiovascular load and, consequently, the metabolic cost of these three jobs were measured in sample subjects by means of an ECG tracing according to Holter methodic. (The results of these tests will not be reported here for the sake of brevity).

The study of alterations of the spine in three different groups of workers was performed using an appropriate questionnaire developed by the authors (Colombini et al.,1986), which was completed for the subjects under study by specially trained nurses. The questionnaire included the following features:
- a detailed working history, aimed especially at identifying previous exposure to occupational risk for the spine;
- separate identification of acute and peculiar manifestations such as discal hernia and acute attacks of lumbago;
- identification of subjects with pronounced chronic spinal disease (cervical, thoracic and lumbosacral) according to established thresholds of severity;
- description of the type and duration of spinal pain and associated factors (disability, sick absence, necessity of treatment);
- confirmation of the diagnoses on the basis of a more extensive clinical-diagnostic protocol used by the authors (Colombini et al.,1986), which in this case supplied data on the control group.

The questionnaire was distributed to the 1157 quarrymen, consisting of 154 caterpillar drivers, 469 sorters, 450 stone cutters and 89 workers doing various other jobs.

In view of the specific aims of this study, the subjects examined were selected according to the following criteria: a) employment on the same job for more than 5 years; b) no previous job involving a risk for the spine lasting more than 4 years. 590 subjects complied with these requirements; they were divided into the three jobs under study and in 4 10-year age classes, as shown in Table 1.

The data on the frequency of chronic spinal disease (cervical, thoracic and lumbosacral) in the three groups of quarrymen and in the corresponding age sub-groups were compared with those already available (Occhipinti et al.,1985) for a control group matched for sex and age. The comparison was made by analysing a series of 2x2 tables and calculating X^2 with Yates correction, the rate ratio and the relative 95% confidence limits. The Rate ratios where the lower confidence limit was ≥ 1 were considered positive (Comba and Axelson, 1981). In addition, in order to overcome the difficulties arising from the low numbers of some job and age sub-groups, and so as to be able to present concise data for each job group, the standardized morbidity ratio (SMR) (indirect standardization) was calculated and the value was confirmed by the X^2 test (Armitage, 1973).

RESULTS AND DISCUSSION
Analysis of Work Postures

A) <u>Caterpillar Driver:</u> the posture is mainly seated with frequent twisting of the trunk due to the need to continually change gear in a confined space; the posture is kept for at least 6-7 hours/day. The driver is subject to shocks and whole-body vibrations on account of the rough terrain (accelerations along the Z axis between 0.10 and 0.30 m/sec^2 for frequencies between 2 and 15 Hz).
B) <u>Sorter</u>: for the whole of the shift, work consists of sorting porphyry slabs (on the ground) using a sledge-hammer or a pickaxe and continually lifting and carrying the slabs (weight 10-35 Kg) to storage pallets (Fig.1). It was estimated that each labourer lifted and carried an average of 250-300 hundred Kg of stone every day. The lumbar loads that develop during these operations vary from 140 to 600 Kg.
C) <u>Stone cutter</u>: the job consists of taking the slab (weight 10-35 Kg) from the storage zone (at a height from the ground of about 1.20 m), with twisting of the trunk; placing the slab under the power hammer (trunk slightly bent, hands stretched away from the body); after cutting, throwing away the cut stones and residual pieces (Fig.1). Each stone cutter handles about 40-80 hundred Kg of stone per day. The resulting lumbar loads that develop vary from 140 to 400 Kg. All workers work on an incentive scheme, which means elevated work rhythms and few pauses.
Without considering the detailed factors, all the jobs studied involved a high risk for the lumbosacral spine: in the caterpillar drivers, because of the seated posture, the trunk torsions and the whole-body vibrations; in the other jobs due to considerably high lumbar loads that develop.

Figure 1. Working postures of sorter and of stonecutter.

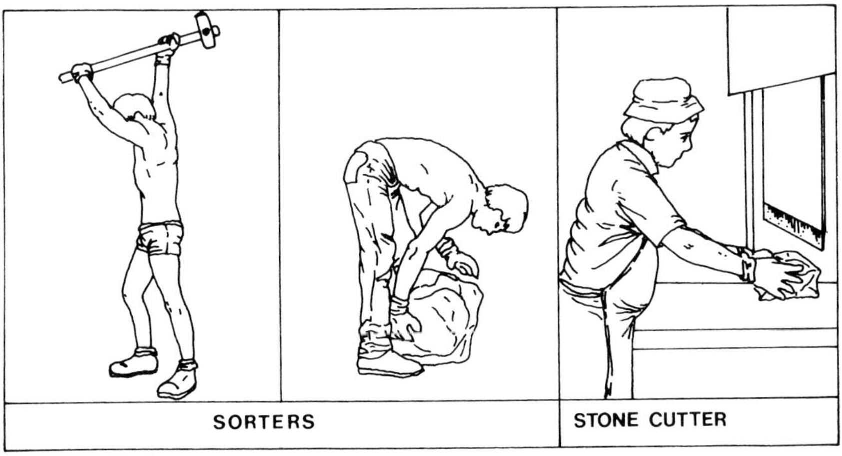

SORTERS | STONE CUTTER

Table 1. Number of subjects examined and mean length of employment in the three groups of quarrymen, by age.

JOB	AGE GROUPS							
	⩽ 25		26-35		36-45		>45	
	N.	len. of empl.(x̄)	N.	len. of empl.(x̄)	N.	len. of empl.(x̄)	N.	len. of empl.(x̄)
Caterpillar Drivers	15	6.8	49	11.4	26	22.6	17	29.5
Sorters	56	6.5	95	9.7	40	15.4	43	28.4
Stone Cutters	46	6.3	75	10.7	36	20.2	92	33.5

Analysis of health data

Only the most significant data obtained from the clinical investigation will be reported here.

Table 2 shows, according to age class and job, the percent frequency of cervical, thoracic and lumbosacral spinal diseases in the three groups of quarrymen studied and in the controls. There was a high incidence of lumbosacral alterations particularly in the younger age classes; conversely, the frequency of thoracic spinal alterations was particularly low in the three groups of quarrymen.

Table 3 analyses the qualitative aspects of the disorders in the three districts of the spine. In particular, for the subjects with segmentary spinal disease, data are reported on: the form in which the disorders occurs (chronic, recurrent), type of disorder (segmentary insufficiency, circumscribed acute pain, diffused pain), whether treatment was required. The number of days of work lost for segmentary disorders, multiplied by 100 subjects at work, is also shown. Attention is drawn to the certainly not negligible figure for days of work lost for lumbosacral disorders in sorters and stone cutters (about one day/year per worker).

The statistical comparisons made (X^2, rate ratio, SMR) confirmed agreement with the data observed in the controls for the various jobs for the cervical and thoracic segments. The situation was exactly the opposite for the lumbosacral segment. The rate ratios were generally significant in the three jobs, compared with the controls, in the two younger age classes; the same degree of significance was not, however, observed in the two older age classes. Nevertheless the SMR (table 4) which shows that there is a general tendency to suffer from lumbosacral disease in each job involving risk, compared to controls, was constantly very high and in any case highly significant from a statistical point of view.

Table 2. Occurrence (%) of cervical (A), thoracic (B), lumbosacral (C) spondyloarthropaty among the three groups examined and among controls, by age.

JOB	AGE GROUPS ≤25	26-35	36-45	≥45	
Caterpillar Drivers	13	16	19	35	(A)
Sorters	7	14	32	26	
Stone Cutters	9	16	28	42	
Controls	12	10	32	40	
Caterpillar Drivers	13	4	0	0	
Sorters	2	2	0	0	
Stone Cutters	7	5	8	3	(B)
Controls	6	4	10	4	
Caterpillar Drivers	47	41	50	53	
Sorters	39	48	45	53	
Stone Cutters	22	23	42	67	(C)
Controls	6	12	28	50	

CONCLUSIONS

Analysis of the work postures in the three main jobs done at the porphyry quarry showed that the lumbosacral segment of the spine was definitely the segment most subject to risk. Parallel health investigations revealed the existence of a significant excess of lumbosacral disease in these groups of workers compared to sex- and age-matched controls. The careful selection of the health data was necessary in order to reduce as far as possible the main confounding variables for the disorder under study, which were age, sex, previous occupational exposure, length of exposure in the specific job. This selection does, however, guarantee greater assurance in making final assessment.

It can therefore be concluded that the porphyry quarrymen contract lumbosacral spinal diseases to a greater extent and at a younger age than in the matched male general population due to the specific working postures.

The only reservation we could have is the fact that we did not find significant rate ratios in the higher age classes. However, these age classes were certainly less represented in the job due to the difficult working conditions,

Table 3. Qualitative aspects of cervical (A), thoracic (B) and lumbosacral (C) disorders; time pattern, type of pain, use of treatment (expressed as a percentage of all cases of cervical spondyloarthropaty); sickness-absence days (n. x 100 workers).

JOB (A)	TIME PATTERN (%) chronic	recurring	TYPE (%) insufficen.	cervic. p.	c. brach.p.	TREAT. (%)	SICKN. ABS days
Caterpillar Drivers	19	81	33	57	10	14	0
Sorters	41	59	17	49	34	34	50
Stone Cutters	42	58	24	48	28	25	94

JOB (B)	TIME PATTERN (%) chronic	recurring	TYPE (%) insufficen,	thoracic p.	TREAT. (%)	SICKN. ABS days
Caterpillar Drivers	25	75	0	100	0	0
Sorters	0	100	0	100	33	17
Stone Cutters	31	69	31	69	31	6

JOB (C)	TIME PATTERN (%) chronic	recurring	TYPE (%) insuffic.	lumbago	sciatica	lum.-scia.	TREAT. (%)	SICKN. ABS days
Caterpillar Drivers	37	63	29	47	2	22	24	13
Sorters	37	63	18	53	0	29	26	118
Stone Cutters	40	60	15	50	3	32	34	106

Table 4. Lumbosacral disorders: SMR and relative significance for each job group as compared with matched control groups.

JOB	STANDARDIZED RATIO OF MORBILITY	
Caterpillar Drivers	217	(P<0.001)
Sorters	230	(P<0.001)
Stone Cutters	153	(P<0.001)

which lead to a high occupational morbidity (silicosis, serious accidents, etc.), so that the workers either change job or continue working at considerably reduced rhythms, work loads (and pay). This selection phenomenon, however, can at the most cause an underestimation of the real incidence of lumbo-sacral spinal disease in these higher age classes; if this is true, the conclusions illustrated above are all the more reliable.

REFERENCES

Armitage, P., 1971, <u>Statistical methods in medical research</u> (Blackwell Scient.Pubbl.)

Colombini, D., Occhipinti, E., Molteni,G., Grieco,A., Pedotti,A., Boccardi,S., Frigo,C., Menoni, O., 1985, Posture analysis, <u>Ergonomics</u>, 28, 95-98

Colombini, D., Occhipinti,E., Grieco, A., Boccardi,S., Menoni, O., 1986, <u>Posture di lavoro e artropatie</u>, 2nd Edn. (Comune di Milano)

Comba, P., Axelson, O., 1981, Ricerche epidemiologiche in Igiene e Medicina del Lavoro, <u>Rapporto ISTISAN n.53</u>

Occhipinti,E., Colombini,D., Menoni,O., Grieco,A., 1985, Alterazioni del rachide in popolazioni lavorative. I: dati su un gruppo maschile di controllo, <u>La Medicina del Lavoro</u> 76, 5, 387-398.

SHOVEL DESIGN AND BACK LOAD
IN DIGGING TRENCHES

Maarten van der GRINTEN

TNO-Institute of Preventive Health Care,
P.O. Box 124,
NL-2300 AC Leiden, The Netherlands

ABSTRACT
    In an experimental field study, the effect of shovel design on back load during digging trenches in compact sand was studied. Three different designs with modestly modified length and curvature of the handle were compared to a "standard shovel." The trunk flexion and the biomechanical moment at L5-S1 were used as parameters of back load. The results showed that a new designed shovel, characterised by a relatively large curvature, is an acceptable alternative to the standard shovel. However, none of the test shovels appeared to be designed in the best possible way for digging tasks in sand with very high thrusting resistance.

INTRODUCTION
    A Dutch municipal drinking-water distribution department employs about 80 workers for installing and maintaining the underground drinking-water pipelines. A considerable part of that work consists of digging and shovelling soil from trenches. In a preliminary study on work and health (Van der Grinten & Poll, 1983) high back morbidity and back load was found within the occupational group and a follow-up program of research and ergonomic, organisational, educational and training actions was suggested.
    The ergonomical follow-up study dealt with recommendations for selecting digging and shovelling tools. More details can be found elsewhere (Van der Grinten, 1986).
    Studies on manual digging and shovelling are known from the beginning of this century and have recently been reviewed by Freivalds (1986a). Most studies concentrate on energy consumption during work. Only one recent study analysed the effect of shovel design on back load (Freivalds, 1986b). In this study compressive forces in the lower back

in "critical postures" were evaluated in two experimental tasks in loose foundry sand with different assembled garden shovels.

In the present experimental study the back load during digging trenches in compact sand is analysed with respect to the use of different shovels. This type of digging in fact consists of two tasks: "digging" and "shovelling". During the digging task a portion of the compact sand is worked loose and thrown away and a portion is lost from the blade. The shovelling task consists of scooping loose sand out of the trench before the next layer is dug away.

Four different shovel designs were used by experienced workers and the effect on back load was analysed.

MATERIALS AND METHODS
Test shovels
Four test shovels were used in this study (Figure 1).

Figure 1. Shovel designs for digging and shovelling sand form trenches.

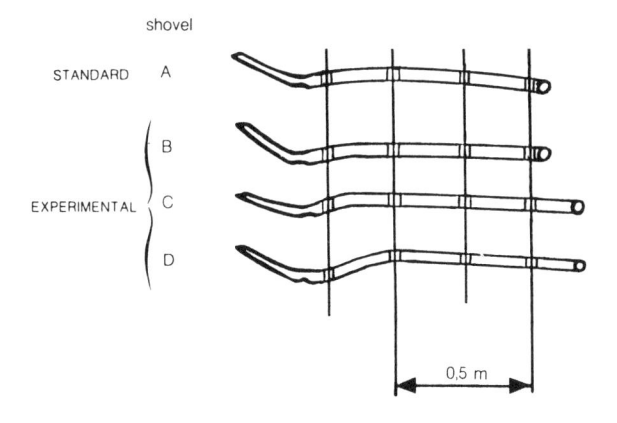

Shovel A is usually purchased by the company ("standard shovel"). Shovel B and C were assembled from commercially available blades and handles and shovel D was a new design. The designs resulted from brainstorming sessions with workers and representatives of shovel manufacturers. It was decided to keep the blade surfaces identical (0.054m²) because sand volume and weight on the blade is more or less controlled by the worker independent of surface size. The major differences between the four shovels deal with length and curvature of the handle.

Field experiments

Six subjects with different body height and working experience as pipe-layer participated in the field experiments on a test location with compact sand. Each subject tested a shovel twice in both tasks (digging and shovelling). To get familiar with the new shovels the subjects used the shovels in practice a few days preceding the experiments. No samples of data were taken at the beginning or end of each trench.

Biomechanical analyses

The working cycle of digging and shovelling consists of four parts: thrusting, lifting, throwing and returning. It is assumed (supported by early results of Lehmann (1933)) that back load is maximum at the beginning of the lifting action. At that instant of the digging cycle, dynamic forces of loosening sand and accelerating the shovel are added to the gravity forces on shovel and trunk. Furthermore, the trunk is in the lowest position near its extreme flexed position.

Working postures and shovel positions at the beginning of the lifting action were registrated with two video camera's. White markers were fixed on the subjects, the shovel handles and a calibration frame. The video pictures were digitized manually, which allowed quantification of the trunk flexion angle and other positional data of the load. Antropometric data were collected and the weight of shovels filled with sand was estimated from samples taken. A simple biomechanical model was used to quantify the biomechanical flexion and twisting moments at L5-S1.

RESULTS

The average trunk flexion and the biomechanical moments at the beginning of the lifting action for each shovel type and each test is shown in figure 2 and 3 respectively.
Shovel D reduced the required flexion significantly in both tasks, 10-14°, compared to the standard shovel A. Shovel B and C showed less reduction. No significant differences in static instantaneous biomechanical moments at L5-S1 have been found. For all shovel types the average biomechanical load was about 200 Nm for digging and 185 Nm for shovelling with average shovel weights of 75 and 50 N, respectively.

Figure 2. Average forward flexion of the trunk at the beginning of the lifting action in digging and shovelling sand from trenches as a function of shovel type.

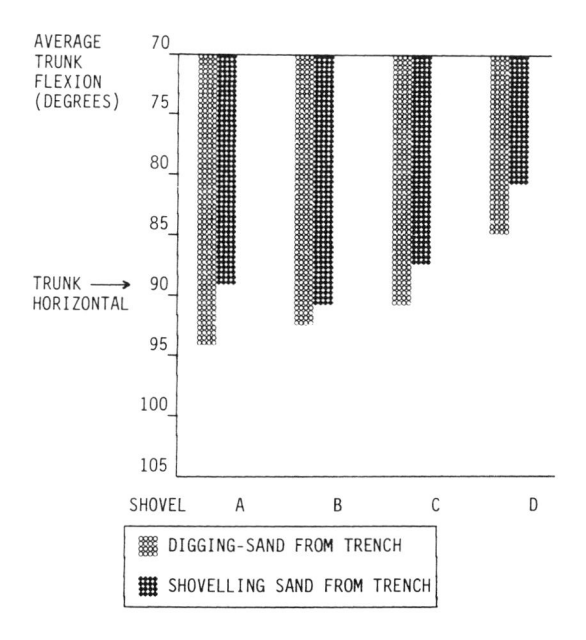

Figure 3. Average biomechanical moments in the lower back at the beginning of the lifting action in digging and shovelling sand from trenches as a function of shovel type.

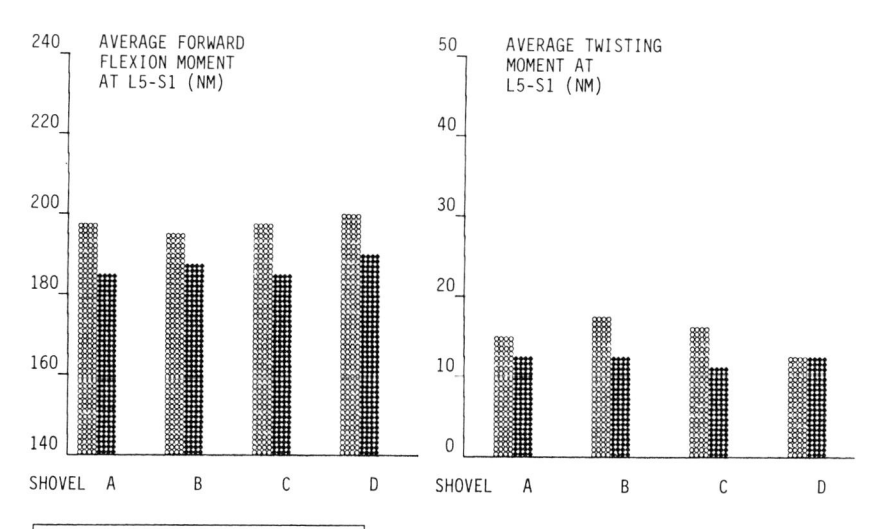

DISCUSSION

Differences in biomechanical load were not found. Reasons for that are of two kinds: (1) the modifications in shovel design were such that increase of moment was avoided as much as possible; (2) the trunk weight contributes about 75% to the biomechanical moment at L5-S1 at the beginning of the lifting action. At that moment the trunk is almost horizontal. Therefore a small reduction of the trunk flexion angle will not result in a great reduction of the instantaneous flexion moments. Nevertheless the small reduction in trunk flexion realised by shovel D can be important for the following reasons:
1. Increase of the "safety margin" towards the extreme flexed position.
2. Reduction of the time spent near extreme flexed working positions in favour of more raised trunk positions.
3. Reduction of time spent in forced flexed postures. When approaching the lowest layer in trenches one shoulder will contact the top of the trench wall due to the flexed trunk. The flexed trunk has to be turned horizontally from a natural digging or shovelling posture to a forced flexed posture parallel to the trench, before flexion between both trench walls can be continued and the lifting action can be started.

In modifying shovel design Freivalds (1986b) changed the lift-angle of the shovel handle to reduce stooping. He found 16° and 32° to be the best angles for shovelling foundry sand. This is in agreement with the lift-angle of 26° designed in shovel D; however apart from the lift-angle stooping was additionally reduced by designing a double bended handle design in shovel D.

In the present paper we have concentrated on the back load during digging and shovelling sand from trenches. The experiences of the participating subjects and work-rates were measured during the experiments as well and used as controlled variables. Data were taken from questionnaires and video-records. It turned out that shovel D rated better or not worse on these aspects in comparison with the other shovels. For these and other tasks as ("shovelling sand under pipes and cables" and "filling in trenches"), shovel D turned out to be a good alternative. However when sand resistance becomes too high and thrusting in the shovel by means of kicking the blade down by foot is no more successful, the whole body weight must be used in leaning over the T-handle; for such purposes all test-shovels should be better designed, especially their handle length.

In this study handle parameters were changed modestly;

if drastically changed without understanding all factors involved, we could have been sure adverse effects would occur. We had such experience when changing the design of a clay shovel and examples are also reported by Freivalds (1986a,b); application of a second handle or a large increase of lift-angle of the handle had adverse effects on the task (loosing sand from the blade) or even the safety of the user (injuring the hand).

CONCLUSION

Taking all back load and other aspects into consideration, shovel D, characterised by a relatively large curvature of the handle turned out to be best, except for sand with very high thrusting resistance; none of the test shovels was designed in the best possible way. It appears that a drastic reduction of back load is not possible by optimising shovel design only. Further reduction of back load is desirable which may be realised by training workers in work-methods. However, mechanisation of this type of work should be considered with first priority.

ACKNOWLEDGEMENTS

This study was initiated and supported by the Drinking-water Distribution Department and partially financed by the Central Personnal Department of the City of Rotterdam. Dr. J. Dul is thanked for his advice.

REFERENCES

FREIVALDS, A., 1986, The ergonomics of shovelling and shovel design - a review of the literature, Ergonomics nr 1, 3-18.
FREIVALDS, A., 1986, The ergonomics of shovelling and shovel design - an experimental study, Ergonomics nr 1, 19-30.
GRINTEN, M.P. van der & K.J. Poll, 1983, Work and Health. A study on health, work and working conditions of the employees in a drinking-water distribution department of the city of Rotterdam (in Dutch). Leiden, NIPG/TNO.
GRINTEN, M.P. van der, 1986, Selection of shovels and spades. Development of recommendations for the selection of tools used in digging and shovelling trenches and holes during installation and maintainance of drinking-water pipe-lines (in Dutch). Leiden, NIPG/TNO.
LEHMANN, G., 1933, Arbeitsphysiologische Werkzeuguntersuchungen, I Die Dynamographie mit Piezoelektrischem Quartz, Arbeitsphysiologie, 6, 640-652.

STATURE CHANGES AND PSYCHOPHYSICAL RATINGS ASSOCIATED WITH REPETITIVE LIFTING

Michael Vincent, Peter Buckle and David Stubbs

Ergonomics Research Unit, Robens Institute,
University of Surrey, U.K.

ABSTRACT

This paper describes an investigation of the effects of repetitive lifting on change in stature and rating of perceived exertion (RPE). Four experimental conditions were studied using 8 male subjects. The mean shrinkage associated with each condition was 3.85mm, 4.76mm, 5.59mm and 7.26mm with increased load being associated with increased height loss. RPE was found to increase with increased load and a significant correlation was found between RPE and height loss. A discussion of the relationship between these variables is presented.

INTRODUCTION

The effect of spinal load may be measured by the extent of visco-elastic compression of the intervertebral discs (Fitzgerald, 1972). The compression of the intervertebral discs and the resulting fluid loss generate a decrease in stature. A number of researchers (Fitzgerald, 1972; Eklund and Corlett, 1984; Tyrell et al, 1985) have shown that changes in stature occur with spinal loading of both a static and of a dynamic nature. Also that a regain of stature can occur following unloading.

As an index of spinal stress, therefore, changes in stature can be used in static and dynamic tasks where the stress will be the result of both the loading and its temporal pattern. In this respect it holds a great advantage over the use of other techniques (see Eklund and Corlett, 1984).

This paper considers the changes in stature and psychophysical ratings (Borg, 1970) with increasing lumbar torque during a repetitive lifting task. Other aspects of the work reported here are described by Vincent (1985).

Materials and Methods

Eight healthy male subjects aged between 22 and 43 years (mean 30.3, s.d. 6.4) with no history of skeletal disorders participated in the study. The mean weight of the subjects was 72.8 kg (s.d. 4.07) and the mean height was 1778 mm (s.d. 48).

Four experimental conditions were considered. These comprised repetitive bimanual lifting of three loads (M1, M2 and M3) whilst standing erect and an additional condition (M0) which involved standing without lifting. A partially balanced experimental design was employed.

The Lifting Task

A repeated lift-hold-relax regime was used, comprising a two second lift, a three second hold, a one second lower and a four second rest. Acceleration was monitored and controlled throughout. A bilateral underhand grip at shoulder width was used to lift from 300mm below shoulder height to shoulder height, at a distance of 435mm (50% of acromion grip length, Pheasant, 1984) from the centre of L5/S1. The acceptable torque on L5/S1 was calculated to be 57.74Nm (M3). Loads relating to 75% and 50% of this value were then derived (43.3Nm (M2) and 28.87Nm (M1) respectively). As lying recovery has been shown to produce a greater regain of stature than standing recovery (Tyrell et al, 1985) a recovery period of forty minutes in the Fowler position was provided at the end of the thirty minute standing recovery period suggested by Tyrell et al (1985) in order to minimise the effects of repeated conditions.

The apparatus and procedures used were similar to those described by Eklund and Corlett (1984).

Procedure

Subjects were asked not to participate in strenuous physical activity on the day before or the morning of the experiment. At 08.58 hrs the subject's stature was measured and at 09.00 hrs the subject began lifting. A clock placed in front of the subject was graduated according to the lift regime described earlier. At the end of each three minute period the subject was asked to stop lifting and stature measurements were made within a two minute period. At the end of the two minute period, the lifting recommenced. The lift/measurement cycle continued for fifty minutes, followed by a thirty minute period of standing and forty minutes in the Fowler position. This constituted a two hour experimental time for each of the four conditions. RPE was recorded at the end of each lifting condition. Aspects of regain in stature whilst standing and in the Fowler position are reported elsewhere (Vincent, 1985).

Results

Figure 1 shows the group means and standard deviations for changes in stature for each of the experimental conditions. Height loss ranged from 3.85mm for M0 to 7.26mm for M3, an increased load being associated with increased height loss. Analysis of variance with time as a covariate and Duncan range procedure showed significant differences ($p<0.05$) between all moments except between M1 and M2.

The mean score and standard deviation (s.d.) for RPE was 6.6 (s.d. 0.7), 9.8 (s.d. 1.5), 11.4 (s.d. 2.3) and 15.1 (s.d. 2.3) for conditions M0, M1, M2 and M3 respectively. Wilcoxon matched-pairs signed-rank test showed all conditions to be significantly different ($p<0.025$). A correlation ($r= 0.519$, $p<0.005$) between RPE and the height loss was observed.

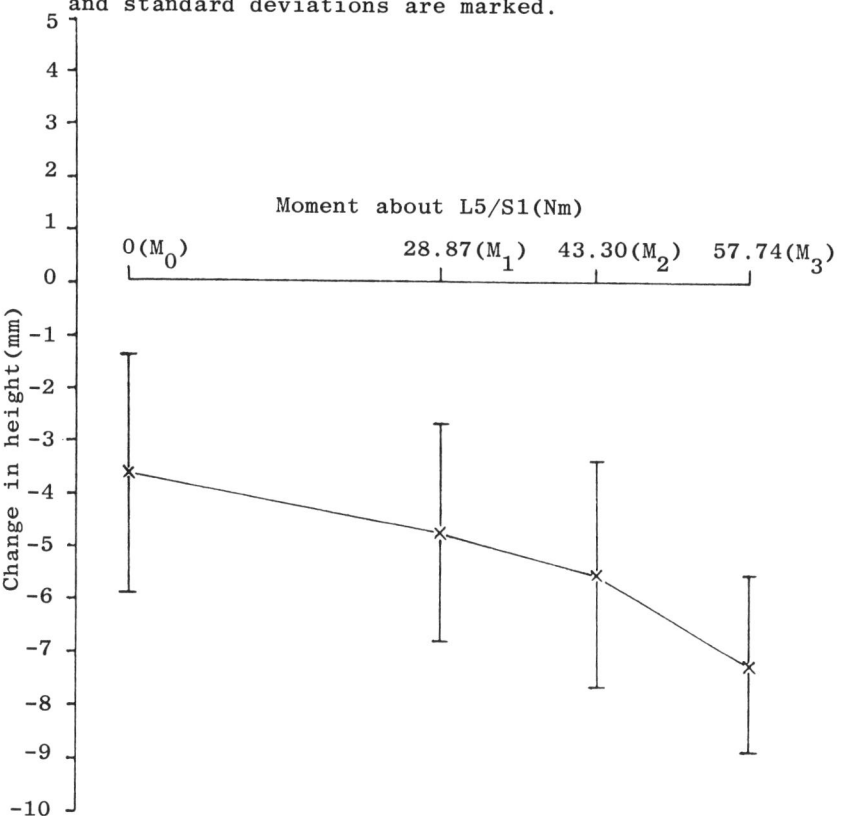

Figure 1. Shrinkage during 50 minutes, with 30 minutes lifting for conditions M_1, M_2, M_3. The group means (n=8) and standard deviations are marked.

Discussion

The mean shrinkage measured for the four conditions was 3.85, 4.76, 5.59 and 7.26mm. Previous studies (Eklund and Corlett, 1984; Fitzgerald, 1972) have shown height losses of between 2 and 4mm/hr whilst standing. The value obtained in this study of 3.85mm may be considered consistent with their findings. The only previous study on repetitive lifting and height loss was undertaken by Tyrrell et al (1985). They demonstrated a mean stature loss of 6.9mm after lifting a 10kg barbell for twenty minutes at a rate of twelve per minute. Comparisons are difficult because of the different rates, duration and styles of lifting involved. However, for approximately the same weight lifted at twice the rate for half the time, the values of 7.26mm and 6.9mm are very similar.

The RPE scale was designed to have a linear relationship with physiological measures and physical workload, the heart rate corresponding to approximately ten times the RPE value. The scores obtained in this study indicate a heart rate of approximately 150 bt min for the heaviest lifting condition. However, Ekblom and Goldberg (1971) have shown that arm exercise gives a higher RPE score at the same heart rate than cycling. RPE may be a better indicator of the task stress associated with the arms than of the trunk, although the two are related.

Whilst a significant correlation was observed between height loss and RPE for this bimanual upright repetitive lifting regime, further studies are required to establish whether this relationship also exists for other postures and force applications. It seems probable that the nature of the task under investigation will be critical in determining the suitability of the use of this technique as an alternative, or complement, to other spinal measures.

Other subjective measures (Vincent, 1985) have also shown weak but significant correlations with change in stature. It would seem that additional biomechanical and physiological effects (e.g. shoulder discomfort) may be more important in determining subjective ratings and RPE than is spinal load alone. The use of these ratings (as reported by Kilbom et al, 1983; Vincent, 1985) for assessing spinal stress should be continued as they have major advantages over many other techniques (e.g. Eklund and Corlett, 1984) in that they need no specialist equipment (which is usually complicated, expensive, relatively immobile and restricting on the subject's movement). The advantages of height loss measurement as a technique for measuring an effect of task stress have already been outlined. The technique does, however, suffer from a number of disadvantages as a high degree of subject co-operation is needed, both postural awareness and control seem to be critical, subjects have to perform the measure with minimal clothing and the worktask has to be interrupted for measurement.

Further research into the effects of age and other individual factors, time of day and 'getting-up' time need to be studied. Research is needed on the cumulative effects of loading and recovery and the relationship between load and rate. Most importantly epidemiological information is needed on the relationship between back pain and height loss data.

REFERENCES

Borg,G.A. (1970) Perceived exertion as an indicator of somatic stress. Scand. J. Rehab. Med. 36, 42-57

Ekblom,B and Goldberg, A.N. (1971) The influence of training and other factors on the subjective rating of perceived exertion. Acta Physiol. Scand. 83, 399-406.

Eklund, J and Corlett, E (1984) Shrinkage as a measure of the effect of the load on the spine. Spine,9,189-194.

Fitzgerald, J. (1972) Changes in spinal stature following brief periods of shoulder loading. Institute of Aviation Medicine. Report No. 514. Farnborough, U.K.

Kilbom, A; Gamberale, F; Persson, J and Annwall, G (1983) Physiological and psychological indices of fatigue during static concentrations. European Journal of Physiology, 50, 179-183.

Tyrell, A ; Reilly, T. and Troup, J. (1985) Circadian variation in stature and the effects of spinal loading. Spine, 10, 161-164.

Vincent, M (1985) An investigation of the relationship between changes in stature and spinal loading. MSc (Ergonomics) Thesis, Univ. of London.

AN EPIDEMIOLOGIC STUDY OF POSTURAL RISK FACTORS FOR SHOULDER DISORDERS IN INDUSTRY

L.J. Fine, L. Punnett, W.M. Keyserling

School of Public Health
University of Michigan
1420 Washington Heights
Ann Arbor, MI 48109   USA

ABSTRACT

In an automobile assembly plant, over a ten month period a prospective case-referent study was conducted. The objective of this study was to determine if non-neutral postures are risk factors for musculoskeletal disorders of the shoulder. The cases consisted of all workers from the four largest departments in the plant who reported to the medical area with complaints of shoulder pain. The referents were randomly selected from all workers from these departments who did not report to the medical area with shoulder or back complaints during this period. During the study, 93 cases and 259 referents were interviewed and examined. Each case was examined on average 49 days (median 28 days) after selection. Of the original referent group, 32% reported at least one episode of shoulder pain in the last year. In addition, each worker's job was filmed in order to characterize the postural and peak force requirements on the shoulder.

On average, these workers spent 24% of the job cycle with the left shoulder at 45 to 90 degrees from the torso and 28% of the job cycle with the right shoulder at the same included angle. Forty-one per cent of all workers were required to work at least briefly during the job cycle with the right shoulder elevated above 90 degrees; the proportion was 35% for the left shoulder. Twenty-seven per cent of all workers were required to elevate both shoulders above 90 degrees during the job cycle. The odds ratios for cases with positive findings on the physical examination were significant for elevation of the left shoulder, right shoulder, and both shoulders (3.2, 2.3 and 4.0 respectively). With increasing proportion of of the job cycle in shoulder elevation there was a significant increase in the odds ratio for each side. In general, the relationships were stronger for the left shoulder than for right shoulder. Peak forces at both the right and left shoulders did not appear to confound these associations. These results may be of assistance in the design of workstation layout and job task sequences.

NECK AND SHOULDER COMPLAINTS AMONG SEWING-MACHINE OPERATORS.
Frequencies and diagnoses in comparison to a control population

S. Blåder, U. Barch Holst, S. Danielsson, E. Ferhm, M. Kalpamaa, M. Leijon, M. Lindh, G. Markhede & B. Mikaelsson

Department of Orthopaedic Surgery, Central Hospital, Borås and the Department of Preventive and Social Medicine, University of Linköping, Sweden

Pain and dysfunction in the neck and shoulder girdle are common complaints in the middle-aged population, but the true prevalence of these complaints is poorly known. Several investigators have found a high frequency among heavy industrial workers and in recent years the interest has also been focused on workers in light mechanical industry. The working conditions of sewing-machine operators (SMO) can be described as "active sitting" with repetetetive arm movements and an unfavourable constrained posture.
During 1984 a multidisciplinary investigation was started to study the frequency of neck and shoulder complaints among a population of sewing-machinists compared with a control population and at the same time study their physical and psychological state of health.

Four textile factories in the western part of Sweden were choosen by help of representants from the Swedish Labour Union. They represented heavy, medium and light production and were economically solid with a low frequency of workers from outside Scandinavia. A questionnaire was sent out to all 224 SMO concerning sociopsychological factors and general health conditions. In addition the questionnaire proposed by the Nordic Council was used to study complaints from the neck and shoulder.
One hundred and ninety-nine SMO answered the questionnaire and whenever needed the questions and answers were translated into Finnish or Serbo-croatian.
One hundred and thirty-one out of 150 women who declared complaints from the neck and shoulder region during the last year participated in a clinical follow-up examination wich was carried out 1-3 months after answering the questionnaire.

The same questionnaire was answered by a matched sample of 280 working women in Linköping in the eastern part of Sweden and 119 participated in the same clinical examination. No diagnosis was made at the time of examination.

The incidence of neck and shoulder complaints during the last year was 75 per cent among the SMO compared to 54 per cent of the controls, wich is statistically significant. No significant difference was found in age distribution between the two groups. The prevalence rate (complaints during the last seven days) was 51 per cent compared to 28 per cent among controls. Approximately one third of the sewing-machinists and controls had had medical attendance or physiotherapy last year. SMO complained more often of daily problems from neck and shoulder and they also had a longer duration of problems. No significant difference in frequency was found between Swedish, Scandinavian and non Scandinavian SMO.

Muscle tenderness in one or several regions around neck and shoulder were common findings but in higher frequency in SMO. The tenderness was often localized to levator scapulae muscle, the trapezius muscle, the muscle origin on the occipital bone and in the paraspinal neck muscles. Background variables for tension syndromes like headache and sleeping problems did not differ between the two groups but tension neck syndrome and humeral tendinitis were significantly more often seen among SMO. Diagnoses of degenerative origin (cervical syndrome and acromioclavicular syndrome) were found in almost the same frequency. In 48 per cent of the SMO and in 64 per cent of the controls the symptoms were too discreet to allow any diagnosis. A high positive correlation between tension neck syndrome and working more than 30 hours a week was found among SMO. This tendency we could not find among the controls. Acromioclavicular syndrome was almost never seen under the age of 50 years.

Our results indicate a relation between the working conditions (constrained posture and "short cycle" movements) of the SMO and complaints from the neck and shoulder.

RSI - THE AUSTRALIAN EXPERIENCE

DR R H MEYER

Chief Medical Officer
Commonwealth Banking Corporation
GPO Box 2719
SYDNEY NSW 2001
AUSTRALIA

Over the last five years, Australia has become the focus of an epidemic of arm pain, predominantly in clerical and keyboard workers. It is regarded in our country as a compensable condition, and costs to industry during this period have run into hundreds of thousands of dollars. Despite the fact that physical signs can almost never be elicited, the condition has been called "Repetition Strain Injury", a term that lends itself to the acronym "RSI". The implications of this label include the assumption that the cluster of symptoms is a physiological entity, that the task is causal (and that therefore the employer is to blame), and that some form of injury has occurred. Not a single one of these assertions has been shown to be true, but in the meantime "RSI" has entered the workers' compensation arena to such an extent that at the present time practically no-one who submits a claim for RSI compensation is refused. In addition, common-law suits are being brought in increasing numbers against employers, with payouts either in or out of court of $50,000 - $100,000 being not unusual.

You will have gathered from all this that there is at last arising in Australia in some circles a healthy and growing scepticism about the whole myth built up around pain in the arm by unions, lawyers, members of the media and, I am embarrassed to say, doctors. In recent months the term "Regional Pain Syndrome" has been suggested, and this is, to my mind, infinitely preferable.

Pain associated with the musculo-skeletal system is by no means new or uncommon, nor is it necessarily restricted to the work environment.

It was referred to by Ramazzini and no doubt has been present since the beginnings of human existence. What is relatively new, though, is the concept of blame, and in Australia this is the axle around which an entire industry revolves. Patients are being treated, usually unsuccessfully, for periods of time which would never be entertained in any other so-called traumatic illness. They are being kept off work for months and years and indeed many will never return to productive work again.

Much has been said about the aetiology of the condition, and two major task force reports were issued in 1985, followed in late 1986 by a "Code of Practice". In gathering material, both committees canvassed a wide area of public opinion and as a result arrived at conclusions which I and many of my colleagues find less than convincing.

It is valid to comment that the weight of opinion among occupational physicians is tending more and more to swing to occupational neurosis as the basic aetiology of the pain suffered by office workers. It is particularly noteworthy that even those occupational physicians who profess not to follow this belief nonetheless treat their patients along largely psychological lines.

It is instructive to reflect that, when speaking of treatments which follow the "physical trauma" school of thought, that is to say physiotherapy, rest, analgesics, splints and occupational therapy, 301 of 809 respondents to the Task Force's "phone-in" found that none had been effective. I have always believed that any treatment regimen boasting a failure rate approaching 40 per cent should be looked at with some scepticism, but the figures appear not to have caused even a minor falter in the unrelenting march of a theory of aetiology that refuses to accept the obvious, but continues to maintain that trauma exists somewhere - "we just haven't found it yet"!

Have a look at the following list. Do the recommendations look familiar? They are almost word for word those that are usually made for preventing arm pains and I agree entirely with them, although I find that they sit strangely with what is purported to be a physical trauma:
a) rational organisation of work-rest schedules for the workers, including introductory or morning gymnastics, the introduction of at least two official work-breaks associated with relaxation exercises;
b) optimal breakdown of the process by phases;
c) alternation of successive operations performed by the same worker;
d) enlargement of tasks;

e) changes in assembly-line speed during the shift;
f) change-over from an assigned assembly timing to a free one;
g) organisation of a rational work tempo and rhythm with an adequate number of micro-pauses;
h) introduction of functional music into the shift schedule;
i) rational workplace design;
j) creation of aesthetic conditions in the working environment which enhance the workers' emotional tonus.

But what they really are, is a series of recommendations to relieve monotony and boredom! ILO (1983)

Perhaps I could illustrate that the psychological approach works by reference to a problem that my bank had a couple of years ago in one of our cheque clearing departments. This was in the early days of the overuse panic, but we were extremely worried by the fact that over quite a short period of time twelve of our operators had been diagnosed as suffering from "repetition strain injury".

I went to the area with one of our industrial relations managers to see what was going on. We started off by interviewing the manager and the supervisors and rapidly reached the conclusion that they were less than sympathetic about the whole situation.

Unfortunately, as we were quick to find out, they communicated their scepticism all too clearly to the operators in the machine room. Matters were not helped by the fact that one of the cases diagnosed as "tenosynovitis" had resigned, mentioning at the same time that she had been pretending symptoms all along!

Next we interviewed the operators themselves, in small groups of four or five, and encouraged them to talk freely.

What came out of our discussions was essentially that morale was low. Most of the operators had joined the bank believing that they would be clerical staff and found themselves as fulltime machinists. All except one expressed a desire to transfer but felt that the chances were minimal - as indeed they were.

Dissatisfaction was also expressed on a number of domestic matters, including location of personal lockers on a different floor, prohibition of eating and drinking in the rest area and alleged unavailability of alternate luncheon room facilities.

A firm policy was introduced laying down the time that operators would have to remain in the department before transfer, and work procedures were changed to provide for stable and predictable hours of duty. The unattractive premises needed upgrading and we recommended that an interior decorator be retained to advise on this aspect to improve the drab, factory-like appearance of the area.

Since then, only two cases have been diagnosed in that department.

In the Australian model, the notion of RSI derives its main support from known medical entities, such as tenosynovitis, carpal tunnel syndrome, de Quervain's tenovaginitis, epicondylitis and even ganglion, with which conditions it is often erroneously equated. These, however, are diagnosed on the basis of both symptoms and physical signs. They recover in the normal course of events. In stark contrast, the RSI seen in over 90% of Australian cases, and particularly those of keyboard operators has no localizing physical signs. Occasionally we see minimal swelling, but this has been described in hysteria for hundreds of years.

We believe that the problem should be looked at as being represented by an "inverted Y":

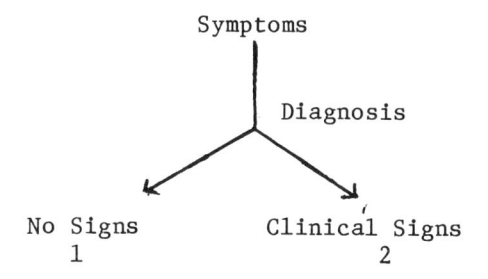

```
           Symptoms
              |
           Diagnosis
          ↙         ↘
    No Signs     Clinical Signs
       1              2
```

In the bank we have never seen a case of "Syndrome 2", nor have we seen documented evidence of keyboard-initiated arm pain's proceeding to a stage where clear physical signs are demonstrated that would lead us to accept a diagnosis of tenosynovitis. We have certainly seen cases of increasing pain and disability, but in none of these have we been able to demonstrate the physical signs that would support such disability.

We believe that the hysteria that has been engendered by well-meaning but misinformed publicity about the dire effects of painful arms has resulted in an epidemic of what has always been called occupational neurosis.

It follows from this that the best, and indeed the only way to combat the condition is to relieve anxiety, create optimum working conditions, and avoid, as far as possible, the aches and pains caused by poor posture, poor ergonomics, poor morale and work overload.

Once the condition is established, patients need reassurance and an early return to work. This work must be of such a nature that pain is avoided, otherwise worry and conflict return and reinforce the original pain. Similarly, it is important that persons who have been absent from keyboard and clerical duties for extended periods be reintroduced gradually to a full workload.

Management of RSI cases in the Commonwealth Banking Corporation

All operators who experience pain or discomfort associated with work activities are encouraged to report to an occupational health nurse or to a supervisor. If possible they are then referred to a doctor at our Occupational Health Division, examined and advised on management. Where the patient is under treatment by a General Practitioner, we ask her approval to discuss the case with her doctor so that we can work together to ensure that when a return to work becomes possible, everything is done to avoid a recurrence. I say "her" because 97 per cent of overuse syndrome in the Corporation occurs in females.

The Commonwealth Bank has over twelve hundred branches all over Australia, so often it is geographically impossible to follow this path. Where distance forbids such close personal supervision, explanatory letters are forwarded to branches, and whenever possible an Occupational Health Nurse visits. If this is not possible due to constraints of distance then every attempt is made to follow-up by telephone.

The most important thing, we believe, is that a patient with pain in the arms be properly diagnosed and if physical signs are absent, that he or she be encouraged to return to some form of work as soon as possible.

Maintenance of good morale is extremely important in both prevention of overuse syndrome and rehabilitation of sufferers, and this is largely a management function. Ergonomically designed furniture is important, but should never be regarded as the final solution in the absence of a supportive and pleasant environment.

We are firmly of the opinion that the painful arm syndrome of clerical workers is real and painful. We are equally as firmly of the opinion that it has its origin in muscle discomfort caused by bad posture and static muscle load. In an environment of low morale, boredom and ill-founded publicity as to possible permanent crippling, the ingredients for an occupational hysteria readily take root.

While the absence of physical signs in an office worker with upper limb discomfort continues to be regarded as a basis for diagnosis of conditions which have traditionally required definite physical criteria, this unfortunate condition will continue to create unhappy "victims". I believe it is time the medical profession began to re-examine the phenomenon of "RSI" objectively in the light of the professional basics in which we have all been brought up to believe.

REFERENCES

International Labour Organization 1983, <u>Encylopaedia of Occupational Health and Safety</u>, 3rd edition.

National Occupational Health and Safety Commission, 1985, <u>Interim Report of the RSI Committee.</u>

National Occupational Health and Safety Commission, 1986, <u>Repetition Strain Injury: A Report and Model Code of Practice</u>

Task Force on Repetition Strain Injury in the Australian Public Service, 1985, <u>Task Force Report.</u>

A REVIEW OF RESEARCH ON REPETITIVE STRAIN INJURIES (RSI)

GABRIELE BAMMER & ILSE BLIGNAULT

Director's Section, Research School of Social Sciences, Australian National University, GPO Box 4, Canberra, ACT 2601 & Early Intervention Unit, Royal Darwin Hospital, PO Box 41326, Casurina, NT 5792, Australia

WHAT ARE RSI?

This review deals with RSI which are work related and which affect the upper body.

Clinically the disorders known as RSI fall into two broad groups: localised and distinct neuro-musculo-tendinous syndromes and more diffuse and ill-defined symptom complexes, apparently muscular, about which little is known. The first group of disorders includes tenosynovitis, rotator cuff syndrome, peritendonitis, epicondylitis and carpal tunnel syndrome. Disorders of the second group may involve single muscles, groups of muscles or more extensive areas. If acute they are often described as muscle strains. Various terms have been used for chronic conditions including occupational myalgia, occupational neurosis, myositis, fibrositis, muscular rheumatism and myofascial syndrome. Two or more of the syndromes may occur concurrently and well-defined syndromes may coexist with diffuse ones.

The pathophysiology underlying RSI is still unclear. Possibilities include mechanical failure; exhaustion of the supply of synovial fluid which lubricates the tendons; local ischemia (oxygen depletion) with concomitant build-up of toxic inflammatory by-products; and energy metabolism disturbance.

Symptoms of RSI include pain, fatigue and weakness in the affected limb or area. Physical signs such as local tenderness, swelling, induration (hardening) or crepitus (a crackling sound when the tendons are lightly pressed) may or may not be present. The most common pattern is, at first, for symptoms to occur only occasionally during work and to be quickly relieved by rest. If no action is taken and the person continues the damaging work, symptoms may become progressively more frequent and persistent, and signs may appear.

ARE RSI NEW?

The more diffuse forms of RSI have been recognised the longest, with the first real acknowledgement being attributed to the Italian, Bernardino Ramazzini, in 1713. He described the disability which can be caused by writers' cramp and since then this problem has been widely reported in the medical literature. In the late 1800s cramps associated with other occupations were also described, most notably among telegraphists and piano players. Most of these reports came from England.

The well-defined forms of RSI such as tenosynovitis seem to have only become common in this century and have been mainly associated with industrial and farm work, although homemakers and tradespeople such as carpenters and upholsterers have also been affected. Reports of these injuries have come from a number of countries.

RSI seem to have been first recognised among office workers in the 1930s, and in the 1950s they became a major problem among keypunch operators in Japan. Since then RSI have been recognised among keyboard operators around the world, with widespread attention being given to this problem since 1980.

ARE RSI COMMON DISORDERS?

It is difficult to compare studies of prevalence and incidence for a number of reasons, one being that different studies measure different disabilities. This is illustrated by some examples:
1) about 50% of Finnish butchers were found to suffer from carpal tunnel syndrome,
2) of a sample of 152 food packers in Finland, 56% were found to have 'muscle-tendon syndrome of the hands and forearms',
3) 37% of data processing operators in one Australian study had hand, wrist and arm pain daily, and
4) among visual display terminal users in the USA, more than 75% had back and neck/shoulder discomfort at least occasionally.

These sorts of prevalence levels are commonly reported. However, there seem to be very few studies which indicate the degree of incapacity (or even pain) suffered by workers in various occupations. This is an area which warrants much further research.

WHAT CAUSES RSI?

There is general agreement that there are 3 main causes of occupationally-induced RSI - rapid repetitive movements, less frequent but more forceful movements, and static loading (ie the work that muscles must do to hold the body or parts of it in certain positions). However, research

Table 1. Factors suggested by the Task Force on Repetition Strain Injury in the Australian Public Service (1985) to influence the incidence of RSI.

ASSOCIATED FACTORS	CHANGE FACTORS
1. FEATURES OF WORK TASK Occupation/kind of work* Physical demands of work* Job design* Design of equipment* Training in use of equipment* Opportunities for rest breaks* Rate of work* Pressure of work*	1. CHANGE IN DEMAND Return to work after a break* Increase in workload* Change in equipment* Reduced tolerance to stress 2. CUMULATIVE EFFECTS Chronic fatigue Response to musculo-skeletal symptoms
2. FEATURES OF WORKPLACE Physical features of workplace* Social context of work	
3. RESPONSE TO WORK AND WORKPLACE Attitudes to the job* Stress responses to work* Method/approach to task*	
4. WORKER CHARACTERISTICS Physical (age*, sex*, level of fitness, associated physical symptoms*) Psychological (personality, anxiety level, emotional reactivity) Work history (years of service*, experience/skill in task*) Life outside work (opportunities for recuperation)	
5. WIDER SOCIAL CONTEXT Cultural attitudes to work Economic factors Attitudes to health and sickness Workers' compensation	

into the factors contributing to these is still in its infancy. For example, out of a long list of possible factors compiled by the Task Force on Repetition Strain Injury in the Australian Public Service in 1985, only 60% (those marked with an asterisk) have been the subject of any empirical investigation (Table 1).

The factors which have been most closely studied are
1) adverse postures and joint positions outside a comfortable mid-range,
2) other work demands, including work load, control over work and job stress, and
3) work organisation, including task specialisation.

There is general agreement that multiple factors are involved, although most studies have only investigated one or a few of these.

HOW CAN RSI BE TREATED?

A number of treatments have been recommended for RSI, although there is some controversy regarding whether they really improve the underlying injury or just alleviate some of the symptoms. Recommended treatments and management strategies include:
- removal from the injury causing work or modifications to that work,
- rest,
- splints or some other form of immobilization of the arm and/or hand,
- drug treatment with the following drugs given singly or in various combinations: analgesics, anti-inflammatory drugs, corticosteroids, sleeping pills, psychotropic medication especially antidepressants and anxiolytics, muscle relaxants, diuretics, local anaesthetics, and vitamin B,
- physiotherapy, especially spray and stretch, ultrasound, cold treatment, heat treatment, diathermy (short wave therapy), massage, manipulation and/or exercises for the injury, hydrotherapy, controlled laser systems, interferential currents, magnetic field therapy, and transcutaneous electric nerve stimulation,
- surgery,
- relaxation, stress management or EMG biofeedback,
- occupational therapy, including home modifications,
- counselling and developing group support systems,
- developing other interests, including exercising healthy parts of the body,
- 'alternative medicine', especially acupuncture and chiropractic.

Two factors are notable in papers on the treatment of RSI. One is their lack of evaluation of the efficacy of the treatments. Studies of the success of various treatment strategies are rare and on the whole are very poor especially with regard to long term follow-up. There has also been no evaluation of differences in efficacy of treatments for different forms of RSI. The second factor is how little treatments have changed since RSI were first described.

It was recognised then, as it is now, that prevention is better than treatment. Again it is worth noting that very few studies have evaluated the effectiveness of prevention strategies.

WHAT ARE THE CONSEQUENCES OF RSI FOR THE INDIVIDUAL?

Numerous case histories make it clear that RSI affect not only the workplace and productivity, but that RSI have considerable impact on all aspects of daily living, and that, for many sufferers, RSI are associated not only with pain and physical disability, but have considerable psychosocial consequences. These include depression, anxiety, marital and family problems, and abuse of alcohol and other drugs. Such problems may be distinct consequences of RSI, for example, depression resulting from chronic pain, or may result from any of the numerous personal, social and economic problems encountered by sufferers.

Despite a wealth of anecdotal evidence, there is a dearth of research on the psychosocial problems associated with RSI.

WHAT HAVE BEEN THE RESPONSES TO RSI?

RSI affect the management of companies employing workers, the government, the legal system, unions, the media and the community. An analysis of how these different groups have responded to RSI would be of great value.

Various government bodies, companies, unions and community health groups have produced literature on RSI, which has generally been of 2 sorts - recognition of the problem and prevention measures. There have been no analyses of these responses. Comparative studies of the role of these agencies in different countries would be useful, as would analyses of their role in bringing RSI to public recognition, their effectiveness in preventing RSI and the impact of their responses on workers. Similarly, the response of the media to RSI remains to be analysed.

The legal system generally becomes involved in RSI

through workers' compensation claims (in some countries only) and through common law actions against employers for damages for negligence. Although there has been little detailed analysis of the effects of different workers' compensation systems on the individual, there is general recognition that some systems (for example those in Australia) place emotional and financial hardship on sufferers and that compensation is commonly inadequate. Some systems are also counter-productive in terms of rehabilitation, not only because of their adversarial nature, but also because they are insensitive to the rehabilitation needs of injured workers, especially women who are unable to claim for child care, household help and so on.

The whole area of responses to RSI is largely unexplored and warrants a much larger research effort.

WHAT ARE THE BROADER ISSUES RELATED TO RSI?

A real understanding of RSI involves consideration of a number of broader, interwoven issues, including the relationship of paid work to other activities, technological change and its effects on both work and work hazards, sex roles, and the functions of the medico-legal system in occupational health and safety. The majority of studies of RSI have not considered such issues at all, and most of those which have, have given them only cursory treatment. There is a need for a detailed analysis of the broader issues relating to RSI and we suggest that the key to prevention lies in the understanding which can be gained from this.

CONCLUSIONS

Although the disorders which are now called RSI have been recognised for centuries, they are poorly understood. There is still no clear picture of what the disorders are, how many people are affected and how seriously, the relative importance of the many factors thought to be involved in causing RSI or how the disorders can best be treated and prevented. While understanding of the medical and psychosocial aspects of RSI is scant enough, there is even less information on the political aspects of the problem. This dearth of knowledge about RSI is in itself a political aspect!

REFERENCES

A bibliography is available from the first author on request.

CARPAL TUNNEL SYNDROME AND ASSOCIATED RISK FACTORS - A REVIEW

James P. Turner and Peter W. Buckle

Ergonomics Research Unit, Robens Institute,
University of Surrey, UK

ABSTRACT

Carpal tunnel syndrome, (CTS), is associated with a number of systemic conditions. This review has also identified many risk factors associated with the condition. These include individual characteristics, states of health and occupational tasks. The relationships between these factors is unclear, as is the underlying pathology. Similarly the current literature does not usually quantify the risk associated with each factor.

INTRODUCTION

At the wrist, the median nerve and the flexor tendons of the fingers and thumb are collectively surrounded by the structures which form the walls of the carpal tunnel. The borders of the carpal tunnel consist of the carpal bones and the transverse carpal ligament.

Carpal tunnel syndrome, (CTS), is a condition characterised by symptoms indicative of focal median nerve dysfunction within the confines of the carpal tunnel. The symptoms include paraesthesia and pain in the regions innervated by the sensory fibres of the median nerve, (distal to the carpal tunnel), and similarly weakness or atrophy of the muscles innervated by its motor fibres. Pain and discomfort in the hand and / or arms may be characteristically accentuated at night.

Electrophysiological tests of median nerve function are necessary to confirm the diagnosis.

Whilst a number of factors are known to be associated with CTS, it is only in recent years that associations between CTS and specific occupational factors have come to light.

THE EXTENT OF THE PROBLEM

Data concerning the annual incidence of CTS in the UK at the moment are currently unavailable. Information about the condition is routinely recorded by government bodies but problems arise in the reporting and classification of the disease. The bulk of our current knowledge about the syndrome comes from the following sources: case studies, studies involving groups of CTS patients, groups of other individuals of whom a proportion were CTS patients and case-control studies.

SYSTEMIC CONDITIONS ASSOCIATED WITH CTS

Acromegaly - Both Yamaguchi et al (1965) and Posch & Marcotte (1976) found that about 0.5% of their groups of CTS patients, (about 1,200 in each case), were acromegalics. CTS appears to suggest ongoing pituitary overactivity, (O'Duffy et al 1973). Treatment of the underlying endocrine disorder, where feasible, appears to relieve the symptoms of CTS.

Amyloidosis - Peri-collagenous amyloidosis appears to predominantly associated with CTS (Bastian 1974; Hallen & Rudin 1966; Hallet 1982; Chapman & Cotter 1982). The last three of these papers refer to case studies refer to case studies involving CTS patients who were treated surgically. Large amorphous masses of amyloid were found in the carpal tunnel and removed at surgery. All these patients were suffering from a form of amyloidosis known as myelomatosis. Other authors refer to microscopic deposits of amyloid present in tissue samples taken at surgery, (Bastian 1974; Bjerrum et al 1984; Lambaird and Hartmann, 1969). No gross masses were evident.

Diabetes Mellitus - About 5 - 8% of certain groups of CTS patients appear to be diabetics, (Phalen 1966; Posch & Marcotte 1976). In another study, Phalen (1970), reports that 16.6% of 379 CTS patients were diabetics. In total 27.2% were either diabetics or had a family history of the disorder. Bell & Clement (1983) refer to a specific case in which the syndrome appeared to be related to the insulin injection site.

Hyperparathyroidism - A few case reports (Firooznia et al 1981; Palma 1983) indicate that hyperparathyroidism whether primary or secondary, (resulting from renal dysfunction), is associated with CTS. In one case, (Firooznia et al 1981), calcium hydroxyapatite was removed from the carpal tunnnel tissues at surgery. Valenta (1975) refers to a case of CTS developing after the removal of a parathyroid adenoma. Subsequent calcification of the bones of the hand was prominent.

Hypothyroidism and Myxoedema - 6.3% of the total of 1,215 CTS patients reviewed by Yamaguchi et al (1965) were also suffering from myxoedema. Treatment of the underlying endocrine condition appears to improve the syndrome (Chisholm 1981).

Renal failure - With the advent of renal dialysis techniques renal patients have been noted to suffer from CTS, (Jain et al 1979; Spertini et al 1984; Halter et al 1981; Warren & Otieno 1975; Delmez et al 1982; Kenzora 1978). Some authors feel that the syndrome is in some way related to the altered haemodynamics resulting from dialysis procedures, (Kenzora 1978; Warren & Otieno 1975). Amyloid deposits are occasionally found at surgery, (Spertini et al 1984; Kenzora 1978)

Rheumatoid arthritis - Yamaguchi et al (1965) and Phalen (1966) report that 7.6-11.2% of CTS patients suffer from Rheumatoid arthritis.

Yamaguchi et al (1965), Phalen (1966) and Posch & Marcotte (1966) present data which suggest that systemic conditions, (such as those mentioned above), account for about 20-30% of the total number of CTS sufferers.

OTHER FACTORS ASSOCIATED WITH CTS

Apart from the systemic conditions mentioned above, the following factors appear to be associated with CTS:

Family History - Gray et al (1979) report a primary familial type of bilateral CTS. Family pedigree suggested an inheritable disorder transmitted by an autosomal dominant gene with a high degree of penetrance. Nineteen, (44%) of the total of 43 living members of the family suffered from the syndrome.

Gynaecological Surgery - Cannon et al (1981) compared 30 workers with CTS with 90 controls. A history of gynaecological surgery (specifically hysterectomy with bilateral oophorectomy) and the use of vibratory hand-held tools were strongly associated with CTS.

Medication - Case studies (Sikka et al 1983; Howard 1982; Clemmensen et al 1984), have been reported in the literature indicating that some drug preparations appear to have precipitated episodes of CTS.

Sabour & Fadel (1970) reports findings concerning 62 women who were diagnosed as suffering from CTS. All were taking oral contraceptive preparations at the time. Their symptoms improved when they stopped taking the 'pill'.

Menopause - Dieck & Kelsey (1985) state that it has generally been felt that women of menopausal age are at an increased risk of developing CTS. In their study 75% of a group of 40 women treated surgically for CTS in a 2 year period were in their fifth decade.

Posch & Marcotte (1976) reports that 7.4% of 1,201 CTS patients were menopausal women.

Occupation - Varying proportions, (34.7-79%), of groups of CTS patients associate their condition with their occupation, (Birkbeck & Beer 1975; Posch & Marcotte 1976; Tountas et al 1983). Repetitive and forceful hand movements, prolonged grasping and pinching and the use of hand held vibratory tools all appear to be implicated, (Punnett et al, 1985; Birkbeck & Beer 1975; Falck & Aarnio 1983 ; Cannon et al 1981; Rothfleisch & Sherman 1978; Jarvinen & Kuorinka 1979; Armstrong & Chaffin 1979).

Pregnancy - Paraesthesia and CTS have been noted to occur in women during pregnancy, (Wilkinson 1960; Wood 1961; Voitk et al 1983). Voitk et al (1983) interviewed and examined 1,000 pregnant women after delivery - 24.5% had experienced symptoms consistent with a diagnosis of CTS during pregnancy. Oedema appeared to be more prominent in those women with hand symptoms.

Premenstrual Syndrome, (PMS) - Dalton (1984) mentions that paraesthesia of the hands and feet is common amongst those women with PMS who also experience water retention and symptoms of weight gain and bloatedness. Although the symptoms may initially be limited to the premenstruum, they may become more severe until present during the whole cycle.

Pyogenic Infections - Case studies of acute episodes of CTS secondary to pyogenic infections of the forearm, (Williams & Geer 1963) and hand (Bailey & Bolton Carter 1955) have been previously reported.

Sex - In the literature female sufferers tend to outnumber male sufferers. In the region of 60-75% of groups of CTS sufferers tend to be females (Tountas et al 1983; Yamaguchi et al 1965; Posch & Marcotte 1976; Birkbeck & Beer 1975).

Trauma (Acute) - 5-6% of the groups of CTS sufferers reviewed by Phalen (1966) and Posch & Marcotte (1976) had previously fractured their affected wrist. Lynch & Lipscomb (1963) reported that of 600 cases of Colles fractures, CTS subsequently developed in 20 wrists, (19 patients). The time lapse between the initial fracture and the symptoms varies, in general from a few hours to a few months.

Vitamin B6 Deficiency - In recent years some studies have suggested that vitamin B6 deficiency might be associated with the development of CTS, (Ellis et al 1976; Ellis et al 1979; Ellis et al 1982; Wolaniuk et al 1983; Hamfelt 1982; D'Souza 1985). There is however no consensus on this at the current time.

CONCLUSIONS AND DISCUSSION

It is evident from the literature that a large number of factors appear to be associated with the syndrome. Unfortunately this paper can only give examples of the more common ones. Systemic conditions appear to be associated with only 20-30% of the total number of cases of CTS. The development of the condition in the majority of sufferers is probably related to other factors.

The underlying physiological mechanisms for the development of the syndrome are not well understood. In some cases inflammatory responses, tissue deposits, tumours and acute trauma appear to account for the syndrome. In the vast majority of cases the picture is less clear.

It is not unreasonable to suppose, therefore, that there might be underlying mechanisms common to many of these associated risk factors. Their identification may lead to a better understanding of the pathology of CTS.

In addition the strengths of association need to be

better established. This would be facilitated by improved routine recording of the presence / absence of the factors mentioned above when patients present with CTS.

ACKNOWLEDGEMENTS

J. Turner is in receipt of a studentship from the Medical Research Council.

REFERENCES

Armstrong, T.J., Chaffin, D.B., 1979, Carpal tunnel syndrome and selected personal attributes, Journal of Occupational Medicine, 21, (7), 481-486

Bailey, D., & Bolton Carter, J.F., 1955, Median nerve palsy associated with acute infections of the hand, Lancet, 268, 530

Bastian, F.O., 1974, Amyloidosis and the carpal tunnel syndrome, The American Journal of Clinical Pathology, 61, 711-17

Bell, D.S.H.,& Clement, R.S., 1983, Reversal of the carpal tunnel syndrome after change of insulin injection sites, Diabetes Care, 6, (2), 211-12

Birkbeck, M.Q., & Beer, T.C., 1975, Occupation in relation to the carpal tunnel syndrome, Rheumatology and Rehabilitation, 14, 218-221

Bjerrum, O.W., Rygaard-Olsen, C., Dahlerup, B., Bang, F.B., Haase, J., Jantzen, E., Overgaard, J.,& Sehested, P.C., 1984, The carpal tunnel syndrome and amyloidosis, a clinical and histological study, Clinical Neurology and Neurosurgery, 86, (1) 29-32

Cannon, L.J., Bernacki, E.J., & Walter, S.D., 1981, Personal and occupational factors associated with carpal tunnel syndrome, Journal of Occupational Medicine, 23, (4), 255-258

Chapman, R.H., & Cotter, F., (1982), The carpal tunnel syndrome and amyloidosis, Clinical Orthopedics and Related Research, 169, 159-162

Chisholm, J.C., 1981, Hypothyroidism: A rare cause of the bilateral carpal tunnel syndrome- A case report and a review of the literature, The Journal of the National Medical Association, 73, (11), 1082-85

Clemmensen, O.J., Olsen, P.Z., & Anderson, K.E., 1984, Thalidomide neurotoxicity, Archives of Dermatology, 120, (3), 338-41

Dalton, K., 1984, The Premenstrual Syndrome and

Progesterone Therapy, 2nd edn (William Heinemann Medical Books, London).
Delmez, J.A., Holtmann, B., Sicard, G.A., Goldberg, A.P., & Harter, H.R., 1982, Peripheral nerve entrapment syndromes in chronic haemodialysis patients, Nephron, 30, (2), 118-23
Dieck, G.S., & Kelsey, J.L., 1985, An epidemiological study of the carpal tunnel syndrome in an adult female population, Preventitive Medicine, 14, 63-9
D'Souza, 1985, Carpal tunnel syndrome: Clinical or neurophysiological diagnosis, (Letter), Lancet, 1, 1104-5
Ellis, J.M., Kishi, T., Azuma, J., & Folkers K., 1976, Vitamin B6 deficiency in patients with a clinical syndrome including the carpal tunnel defect. Biochemical and clinical responses to therapy with pyridoxine, Research Communications in Chemical Pathology and Pharmacology, 13, (4), 743-57
Ellis, J.M., Folkers, K., Wanatabe, T., Kaji, M., Saji, S., Caldwell, J.W., Temple, C.A., & Wood, F.S., 1979, Clinical results of a cross-over treatment with pyridoxine and placebo of the carpal tunnel syndrome, The American Journal of Clinical Nutrition, 32, (10), 2040-46
Ellis, J.M., Folkers, K., Levy, M., Shizukuishi, S., Lewandowski, J., Nishii, S., Schubert, H.A., & Urlich, R., 1982, Response of Vitamin B6 deficiency and the Carpal tunnel syndrome to Pyridoxine, Proceedings of the National Academy of Science, (USA), 79, 7494-98
Falck, B., & Aarnio, P., 1983, Left-sided carpal tunnel syndrome in butchers, Scandinavian Journal of Work and Environmental Health, 9, 291-297
Firooznia, H., Golimbu, C., & Rafii, M., 1981, Carpal tunnel syndrome as an effect secondary to hyperparathyroidism, Archives of Internal Medicine, 141, 959
Gray, R.G., Poppo, M.J., & Gottlieb, N.L., 1979, Primary familial carpal tunnel syndrome, Annals of Internal Medicine, 91, 37-40
Hallen, J., & Rudin, R., 1966, Peri-collagenous amyloidosis, a study of 51 cases, Acta Medica Scandinavica, 179, (4), 483-99
Hallet, J., 1982, Tendon tethering in the carpal tunnel syndrome in Bence-Jones myelomatosis, The Journal of Bone and Joint Surgery, 64B (3),357-60
Halter, S.K., DeLisa, J.A., Scardapane, D., & Sherrard, D.J., 1981, Carpal tunnel syndrome in chronic renal dialysis patients, Archives of Physical Medicine and

Rehabilitation, 62, (5), 197-201

Hamfelt, A., 1982, Carpal tunnel syndrome and vitamin B6 deficiency, Clinical Chemistry, 28, (4), 721

Howard, J.F., 1982, Arthritis and carpal tunnel syndrome associated with disulfiram, (antabuse), therapy, Arthritis and Rheumatism, 25, (12), 1494-96

Jain, V.K., Rafael, R.V., Cestero, V.M., & Baum, J., 1979, Carpal tunnel syndrome in patients undergoing maintenance hemodialysis, The Journal of the American Medical Association, 242, (26), 2868-69

Jarvinen, T., & Kuorinka, I., 1979, Prevalence of tenosynovitis and other occupational injuries of upper extremities in repetitive work, Arh. Hig. Rada. Toksikol., 30,1281-1284

Kenzora, J.E., 1978, Dialysis carpal tunnel syndrome, Orthopedics 1, (3), 195-203

Lambaird, P.A., & Hartmann, W.H., 1969, Hereditary amyloidosis, the flexor retinaculum and carpal tunnel syndrome, American Journal of Clinical Pathology, 52, (6), 714-19

Lynch, A.C., & Lipscomb, P.R., 1963, The carpal tunnel syndrome and Colles' fractures, Journal of the American Medical Association, 185, (5), 363-366

O'Duffy, J.D., Randall, R.V., & MacCarty, C.S., 1973, Median neuropathy, (carpal tunnel syndrome), in acromegaly, a sign of endocrine overactivity, Annals of Internal Medicine, 78, 379-383

Palma, G., 1983, Carpal tunnel syndrome and hyperparathyroidism, Annals of Neurology, 14, (5), 592

Phalen, G.S., 1966, The carpal tunnel syndrome - Seventeen years experience in diagnosis and treatment of 654 hands, The Journal of Bone and Joint Surgery, 48-A, (2), 211-228

Phalen, G.S., 1970, Reflections on 21 years' experience with the carpal tunnel syndrome, Journal of the American Medical Association, 212, (8), 1365-1367

Posch, J.L., & Marcotte, D.R., 1976, Carpal tunnel syndrome - An analysis of 1,201 cases, Orthopaedic Review, 5, (5), 25-35

Punnett, L., Robins,J.M., Wegman, D.H., & Monroe Keyserling, W., 1985, Soft tissue disorders in the upper limbs of female garment workers, Scandinavian Journal of Environmental Health, 11, 417-425

Rothfleisch, S., & Sherman, D., 1978, Carpal tunnel syndrome, Biomechanical aspects of occupational occurrence and implications regarding surgical management, Orthopaedic Review, 7, (6), 107-109

Sabour, M.S., & Fadel, H.E., 1970, The carpal tunnel syndrome- a new complication ascribed to the pill, American Journal of Obstetrics and Gynecology, 107, (8), 1265-67

Sikka, A., Kemmann, E., Vrablik, R.M., & Grossmann, L., 1983, Carpal tunnel syndrome in association with danazol therapy, The American Journal of Obstetrics and Gynecology, 147, (1), 102-103

Spertini, F., Wauters, J.P., & Poulenas, I., 1984, Carpal tunnel syndrome: A frequent invalidating, long-term complication of chronic haemodialysis, Clinical Nephrology, 21, (2), 98-101

Tountas, C.P., MacDonald, C.J., Meyerhoff, J.D., & Bihrle, D.M., 1983, Carpal tunnel syndrome, a review of 507 patients, Minnesota Medicine, Aug, 479-482

Valenta, L.J., 1975, Hyperparathyroidism due to parathyroid adenoma and carpal tunnel syndrome, The Annals of Internal Medicine, 82, (4), 541-42

Voitk, A.J., Mueller, J.C., Farlinger, & D.E., Johnston, R.U., 1983, Carpal tunnel syndrome in pregnancy, The Canadian Medical Association Journal, 128, (3), 277-81

Warren, D.J., & Otieno, L.S., 1975, Carpal tunnel syndrome in patients on intermittent haemodialysis, The Postgraduate Medical Journal, 51, 450-52

Wilkinson, M., 1960, The carpal tunnel syndrome in pregnancy, The Procedings of the National Academy of Science, (USA), 79, 7494-7498

Williams, L.F., & Geer, T., 1963, Acute carpal tunnel syndrome secondary to pyogenic infection, The Journal of the American Medical Association, 185, (5), 409-10

Wolaniuk, A., Vadhanavikit, S., & Folkers, K., 1983, Electromyographic data differentiates patients with carpal tunnel syndrome when double blindly treated with pyridoxine and placebo, Research Communications in Chemical Pathology and Pharmacology, 41, (3), 501-11

Wood, C., 1961, Paraesthesia of the hand in pregnancy, British Medical Journal, 2, 680-82

Yamaguchi, D.M., Lipscomb, P.R., & Soule, E.H., 1965, Carpal tunnel syndrome, Minnesota Medicine, Jan, 22-33

CONSERVATIVE MANAGEMENT OF
CARPAL TUNNEL SYNDROME
UTILIZING PYRIDOXINE

Morton L. Kasdan, M.D., F.A.C.S.

4006 Dupont Circle
P. O. Box 6048
Louisville, Kentucky 40206

INTRODUCTION
The busy hand surgeon will hear complaints from patients of pain, numbness, tingling, and weakness which are commonly associated with median nerve irritation at the wrist. This symptom complex is usually referred to as carpal tunnel syndrome (CTS). It was generally accepted for many years that the only satisfactory method of treatment was surgery (Bergfield et al., 1983; Graham, 1983; Phalen, 1966; Sakellarides, 1983, Yamaguchi et al., 1965). Surgery will treat the symptoms, but does not correct the etiology of CTS. Even after decompression of the carpal tunnel and relief of symptoms, the patient is usually restricted from a job requiring the use of rapid repetitive gripping tools and/or pinching activities. After learning of the work of Ellis (Ellis et al, 1977; Ellis et al., 1979; Ellis et al., 1981; Ellis et al., 1979; Folkers et al., 1978), this author developed a protocol for the conservative management of CTS. This consisted of the treatment of any pre-existing systemic disease, modification of activities, wrist splints to be worn during sleep, and 200 mgs. of vitamin B-6 a day.

METHODS AND MATERIALS
The medical records of 1122 patients (1673 hands) were reviewed between 1973 and 1985. These patients presented with a classic history and physical findings compatible with a diagnosis of CTS. The definitive diagnosis was based on history, physical examination, and electrical diagnostic studies. The physical examination was considered diagnostic for CTS if two of three findings were present: a positive Tinel's sign, Phalen's test, or obvious thenar atrophy. The electrical diagnostic studies

were performed by a neurologist. A neurological evaluation was obtained at the time of the nerve conduction studies and EMG. A sensory latency longer than 3.4 or 0.3 longer than the opposite median nerve measurement or a comparative measurement of the ulnar nerve on the same hand was considered abnormal. The motor latency longer than 4.0 or 1.0 longer than the opposite hand measurement or comparative measurement of the ipsilateral ulnar nerve was determined abnormal (Felsenthal, 1977; Kim, 1983; Spindler & Dellon, 1982; Thomas et al., 1967).

Before we began using Pyridoxine, the conservative treatment of carpal tunnel syndrome consisted of wrist splints in the neutral position, the use of nonsteroidal anti-inflammatory agents, and a job or activity change. Some patients received steroid injections.

After reading the reports of Ellis and others utilizing Pyridoxine (Ellis et al., 1977; Ellis et al., 1979; Ellis, et al., 1981; Ellis et al., 1979; Folkers et al., 1978; Shizukuishi et al., 1980; Wolaniuk et al., 1983), we began in 1980 to add this to our regimen of management. We have found that patient compliance is best with 100 mgs. of vitamin B-6 twice a day. When the patient notices a relief of symptoms and the condition appears stable, the vitamin B-6 is reduced to 100 mgs. per day.

RESULTS

Of the 1122 (1673 hands) patients examined, 96 patients (126 hands) had a final diagnosis other than carpal tunnel syndrome. The final diagnosis was based on the neurological examination and further testing.

Seven of the 1122 patients studied (8 hands) had acute, traumatic carpal tunnel syndrome. In six of these patients (six hands), the median nerve was decompressed as the presenting injury was repaired.

Six hundred sixteen of the 808 patients with a recorded Phalen's test had a positive result (923 of 1297 hands). Four hundred twenty-eight patients (641 hands), of a total 802 patients (1199 hands) with a recorded Tinel's, had positive tests. The mean age of patients with a final diagnosis of carpal tunnel syndrome (1026 patients, 1547 hands) was 42 years. Patients ranged in age from 17 to 86. There were 570 female and 456 male patients. It is generally found that carpal tunnel syndrome occurs more often in women than men. The common ratios are from 2:1 to 4:1 (Bergfield et al., 1983; Graham, 1983; Phalen, 1966, 1970; Sakellarides, 1983; Yamaguchi et al., 1965).

The most common associated conditions found were

osteoarthritis and obesity. Approximately 31% (318) of the patients with a final diagnosis of CTS had a history of osteoarthritis. This was found most often in the hands, wrists, or cervical spine. Obesity was a problem in 302 patients or 29.4%.

Symptoms during pregnancy were reported by 14 of the 570 female patients; complete resolution of symptoms was reported by four postpartum. A large number of female patients had a history of a hysterectomy and/or oophorectomy. As many patients were uncertain as to the distinction between the two, a final determination was difficult. The use of oral contraceptives was admitted by only 16 female patients.

Symptoms were attributed to occupation by 407 patients. Thirty-two directly related symptoms to an injury on the job. Nocturnal pain was reported by 986 patients.

TREATMENT

Prior to 1980, our overall success with the various forms of conservative treatment used; wrist splints, job changes, anti-inflammatory agents, and steroid injections; was 14.3%. Surgical decompression of the carpal tunnel was performed on approximately 20% of the 147 patients so treated. Forty-two per cent had little or no alleviation of symptoms with conservative treatment, but did not desire surgery. Full, long-term alleviation of symptoms was obtained by four of the 72 hands receiving steroid injections. The average length of follow-up in these patients was 13 months. The remaining patients were lost to follow-up.

Of the 526 patients (768 hands) treated using Pyridoxine, either alone or with wrist splints and/or a job change, 68% (358 patients, 533 hands) had a full or satisfactory alleviation of symptoms. A case was considered to have relief of symptoms if the patient had no nocturnal symptoms and only occasional finger tingling during the day. In more severe cases, an improvement may be seen in the initial three months, but a good alleviation of symptoms will often require longer. Usually patients will respond (if they are going to) in three months.

Surgery for decompression of the carpal tunnel was performed on 328 hands (279 patients) or 27% of the 1026 CTS cases. Forty-nine of the 279 surgery cases (73 hands) had incomplete records due to less than three months follow-up. There was patient satisfaction for relief of symptoms in approximately 97% of the remaining surgically treated cases. In 23 cases (10%), there was a recurrence of some symptoms after an initially good postoperative response. These recurrences were often related to a change of job or activities, symptoms usually cleared upon cessation of the aggravating activity. Only one patient required a second surgical procedure. The remaining cases had a fair result with some alleviation of symptoms or were lost to follow-up.

DISCUSSION

It is felt by many that a diagnosis of carpal tunnel syndrome can be made based strictly on clinical examination (Phalen, 1966, 1972). There are a number of disorders with symptoms similar to those found in carpal tunnel syndrome which may also have a positive Phalen's or Tinel's test. Thorough neurological evaluation and further diagnostic testing are necessary for a positive diagnosis. We have found, as did Phalen, that a wrist flexion test can be negative in advanced cases of carpal tunnel syndrome (Phalen, 1966). Motor and sensory latency testing is also helpful for an objective examination in cases which involve compensation where symptoms are often exaggerated. A neurological consultation is helpful in determining if there are any underlying disorders which are contributing to the problem.

Approximately 40% of our patients had occupations involving the use of tools requiring repetitive use of the hands. Occupation is a factor in carpal tunnel syndrome in this and other studies (Rothfleisch & Sherman, 1978; Bernacki et al., 1981). There is some argument that patients have a predisposition to carpal tunnel syndrome that is aggravated by their occupation (Armstrong & Chaffin, 1979; Bernacki et et al., 1981). We feel this is true, especially in postmenopausal women and women who have had gynecological surgery.

We had little success with conservative treatment of patients with CTS in the earlier years of this study. Unlike Gelberman and Phalen (Gelberman et al., 1980; Phalen, 1966), who have had some success with steroid injections in 22-24%, we found, as did others, 85-95% of the patients injected ultimately had a recurrence of symptoms (Bergfield et al., 1983; Crow, 1960; Foster, 1960; Goodwill, 1965). Steroid injections are used very little in treating carpal tunnel syndrome due to our lack of long-term success with the procedure and an increasing reluctance on the part of our patients to receive injections of steroids. Some authors report little success with the use of Pyridoxine in the treatment of CTS. There

have been reports that as many as two-thirds of the
patients with carpal tunnel syndrome require surgery (Smith
et al., 1984; Byers et al., 1984; Amadio, 1985). We have
been pleased with our results and currently use B-6 to
treat the majority of our patients. There has been some
question as to the danger of using B-6 in high dosages
(Schaumburg et al., 1983). These reports usually site
megadoses of two grams or more. Our patients received a
maximum of 200 mgs. a day. We do caution our patients that
Pyridoxine can be dangerous if taken in excess.

REFERENCES

Amadio, P., 1985, Journal of Hand Surgery, 10, 237.
Armstrong, T. & Chaffin, D., 1979, Journal of Occupational Medicine, 21, 481.
Bergfield, T., Aulicino, P. & Depuy, T., 1983, Orthopedic Review, 12, 5.
Bernacki, E., Walter, S. & Cannon, L., 1981, Journal of Occupational Medicine, 23, 255.
Byers, C., Delisa, J., Frankel, D., & Kraft, G., 1984, Archives of Physical Medicine and Rehabilitation, 65, 712.
Crow, R., 1960, British Journal of Medicine, 1, 1611.
Ellis, J., Azume, J., Tatsuo, W., & Folkers, K., 1977, Research Communication in Chemical Pathology, and Pharmacology, 17, 175.
Ellis, J., Kishi, T., Azuma, J., & Folkers, K., 1979, Research Communication in Chemical Pathology, and Pharmacology, 13, 743.
Ellis, J., Folkers, K., Levy, M., Takemura, K., Shizukuish, S., Ulrich, R., & Harrison, P., 1981, Research Communication in Chemical Pathology, and Pharmacology, 33, 331.
Ellis, J., Folkers, K., Watanabe, T., Kaji, M., Seisuke, S., Cadwell, J., Temple, C., & Wood, F., 1979, American Journal of Clinical Nutrition, 32, 2040.
Folkers, K., Ellis, J., Watanabe, T., Sajii, S., & Kaji, M., 1978, Proceedings of the National Academy of Sciences U.S.A., 75, 3410.
Foster, J., 1960, Lancet, 1, 454.
Gelberman, R., Aronson, D. & Weisman, M., 1980, Journal of Bone and Joint Surgery (Am), 62, 1181.
Goodwill, C., 1965, Annals of Physical Medicine.
Graham, R., 1983, Orthopedics, 6, 1283.
Kim, L., 1983, Orthopedic Review, 12, 59.
Phalen, G., 1972, Clinical Orthopaedics and Related Research, 83, 29.

Phalen, G., 1966, Journal of Bone and Joint Surgery (Am), 48(A), 211.
Phalen, G., 1970, Journal American Medical Association, 212, 1365.
Rothfleisch, S. & Sherman, D., 1978, Orthopedic Review, 7, 107.
Sakellarides, H., 1983, Orthopedic Review, 12, 77.
Schaumburg, H., Kaplan, J., Windebank, A., Nicholas, V., Stephan, R., Pleasure, D. & Brown, M., 1983, New England Journal of Medicine, 309, 446.
Shizukuishi, S., Nishii, S., Ellis, J. & Folkers, K., 1980, Biochemical and Biophysical Research Communication, 95, 1126.
Smith, G., Rudge, J. & Peters, T., 1984, Annals of Neurology, 15, 104.
Spindler, H. & Dellon, A., 1982, Journal of Hand Surgery, 7, 260.
Thomas, J., Lambert, E. & Cseuz, K., 1967, Archives of Neurology, 16, 635.
Wolaniuk, A., Vadhanavikit, S. & Folkers, K., 1983, Research Communication in Chemical Pathology & Pharmacology, 41, 501.
Yamaguchi, D., Lipscome, P. & Soule, E., 1965, Minnesota Medicine, 48, 22.

A NATIONAL STRATEGY FOR THE PREVENTION AND MANAGEMENT OF RSI

Ms K Liddicoat and Dr N Ellis

Worksafe Australia
GPO Box 58, Sydney, 2001

Repetition Strain Injury (RSI) is an occupational health issue that has generated much controversy and confusion in Australia. Its rising incidence during the 1980s, particularly among keyboard workers, caused considerable concern throughout the community and attracted wide publicity. Its significance as a major occupational health issue was reflected by the fact that it was one of two topics given top priority for investigation by the National Occupational Health and Safety Commission - Worksafe Australia.

This paper will describe the Australian Experience of RSI and the development of a National Strategy for prevention and management.

It will include a report on the decrease in incidence in some sectors of the workplace and the development of a description considered more appropriate to the condition, reflecting a shift in emphasis from the medical/biomechanical approach, to one which accommodates psychosocial processes and other influences in the workplace.

The background to the strategy provided in the paper has been drawn largely from Worksafe Australia's Repetition Strain Injury A Report and Model Code of Practice.

At the outset, a short history of the current incidence of the condition in the Australian workplace will be provided as a backdrop to the strategy.

Background Statistics

From 1979-80 Workers Compensation statistics indicated an alarming upward trend in the reporting of the condition in both the blue and white collar sectors and in one State - New South Wales, the condition was a more serious problem for women (1).

Again in New South Wales in the 1980's, industry details revealed the largest number of cases occuring in the industry groups "metals machinery manufacturing" with a significant growth rate in the number of cases reported each year occurring in the industry group "professional" which included clerical and administrative staff (2).

At this point, I will attempt to identify the condition under study and I assure you that debate on this issue continues.

The type of disease appearing on workers' compensation claim forms is coded according to the Ninth Revision of the International Classification of Diseases (ICD-9). The ICD categories of particular relevance to RSI are Code 726 (Peripheral enthesopathies and allied syndromes) and Code 727 (Other disorders of synovium, tendon and bursa). However, ICD-9 does not make specific provision for the coding of RSI, and consequently some RSI cases are likely to be coded to other ICD categories. This problem has been compounded by variations in the medical diagnosis of RSI, and in coding procedures. One State - South Australia, recently introduced a new category in the type of accident classification to flag RSI cases (3).

Unfortunately ICD-9 codes do not identify the cause (i.e. overuse) and therefore some cases reported in statistics may not be relevant. Similarly, we believe some cases may have been coded under other ICD cadegories.

The definition, description and management of the condition will be further developed later in the paper.

The Literature

A number of literature reviews have demonstrated that the condition or similar musculo-skeletal conditions, have been the subject of investigation and concern by researchers and practitioners in occupational health and safety in Australia and overseas for many years, however, it was not until the early 1980's that what we called RSI had become a public issue.

The National Occupational Health and Safety Commission, in its publication, Repetition Strain Injury A Report and Model Code of Practice (1986) presented an international overview of conditions closely resembling RSI.

The review began by citing Ramazzini, who in 1700 recognised that posture and movement at work can affect health, with our attention being drawn to the particular case of scribes.

"Furthermore, incessant driving the pen over paper causes intense fatigue of the hand and the whole arm because of the continuous and almost tonic strain on the muscles and tendons, which in course of time results in failure of power in the right hand "(4).

In our investigations we have found a wide variety of terms in other countries to describe the condition known in Australia as RSI. We consider that this has hampered comparative research, based on international data into the nature and distribution in the population of RSI, and has probably contributed to the widespread belief in Australia that RSI is a uniquely Australian condition (5).

A term used often overseas with wide acceptance is Occupational Cervico-Brachial Disorder (OCD) being present in literature in Japan and the Scandinavian countries.

However, other countries are different because of differences in methods of recording cases of occupational injury and disease and systems of workers compensation (6).

Individual Countries
The following countries have contributed significantly to the pool of knowledge on musculo-skeletal injuries at work, Sweden, Japan, Norway and the United States. Worksafe Australia's Report of May 1986 gives details of their investigations.

The Australian Experience
International activities notwithstanding, there has been a strong and substantial body of opinion within Australia which unfortunately, has served to influence debate on the nature of the condition. This debate has

often taken place in the media and given distorted representation of opinions and data. As a consequence, these actions have caused distress to those with the condition and impeded those attempting to implement prevention strategies (7).

The *Interim Report of the RSI Committee* provided detail of the Australian experience of RSI, past and present. This information received significant praise as a valuable contribution to the understanding of the background to the present situation.

In May of 1986 several major papers were published in the Australian medical literature. 39 research projects on RSI either underway or about to commence were identified. A review of this information was undertaken and a statement of the current knowledge was given in the Commission's final report.

WELL-DEFINED CONDITIONS

There is long-standing evidence in the scientific literature and widespread acceptance that work involving one or more of the following - repetitious tasks, forceful movements and the maintenance of constrained postures for prolonged periods - may be associated with a number of well-defined clinical conditions for which there are accepted means of diagnosis. The mechanisms of these well-defined conditions, however, are not always known. Rotator cuff syndrome, lateral and medial epicondylitis, carpal tunnel syndrome and tenosynovitis are examples of such conditions.

POORLY-DEFINED CONDITIONS

There appears to be agreement that the majority of cases of RSI do fall into this category. The most notable feature of the majority of cases is the reporting of pain in the upper limb or neck.

Theory of Muscular Origin

There is a body of medical opinion that these conditions are accompanied by subjective signs such as tenderness, loss of power and loss of movement, which (along with the history of pain) are reproducible and consistent, enabling this category of RSI also to be considered a distinct clinical entity, of as yet unknown pathogenesis but probably of muscular origin.

This body of opinion recognises that psychological complications are a common feature of this condition and attributes them to:

    the effect of chronic pain and disability;

    less frequently, the adversary nature of the medico-legal process of workers' compensation.

Descriptions of a series of cases by treating medical practitioners support this argument. In the past, preliminary histopathological and electromyographical investigation of muscle tissue has been done, but the results have not been conclusive and, until further work is undertaken, this will not be confirmed.

Theory of Nervous and Vascular Systems Involvement
Other bodies of medical opinion hold that these conditions may be due to mechanisms involving the autonomic nervous system, the brachial plexus, cervical nerve roots, the lesser-known peripheral pain pathways and the vascular system. These models are less developed and, as yet, largely unsubstantiated.

Opposing bodies of opinion hold that this poorly-defined condition is not due to tissue pathology in the upper limb or neck but to psychological processes entirely, and may be broadly divided into two camps (outlined below), although there tends to be a spectrum of opinion in between.

Theory of Work Stress
The use of psycho-metric screening tools in some studies in Australia has revealed that keyboard operators with RSI are more likely to report lack of autonomy, increased work pressure, difficulties with interpersonal relationships at work, depression, as well as complaints about the physical working environment and pain and stiffness at work. Although it is not possible to determine whether the psycho-social factors are a cause of RSI or a result of RSI, it has been postulated that this is evidence that stress at work, due to poor work organisation and job design resulting in monotonous jobs requiring high levels of concentration with little autonomy, contribute to the onset of RSI (8).

This view is supported in a recent article by a sociologist Evan Willis, which describes RSI as a socio-political process to resist dehumanisation of work.

Theory of Psychiatric Disorders
Another opinion that has been expressed is that the poorly-defined version of RSI is a conversion disorder; that is, a conflict exists either at work or privately which is resolved by adopting symptoms which also allow support to be gained from the environment. This theory has not been substantiated.

Combination
The view taken by some organisations with effective RSI prevention strategies in place appears to include components of both the physical and psycho-social models, and is that this condition is likely to commence with discomfort, assumed to be as a result of muscle fatigue resulting from work. Psycho-social factors are then considered important in the progression of this condition to a chronic, disabling painful syndrome; dissatisfaction with, or pressure at, work and fear of sustaining a crippling permanent condition are thought to be important.

It is fortunate that whatever model of causation is adopted, the recommended method of prevention and management is the same. All sources of opinion appear to agree that the condition should be taken seriously by management and actions determined in consultation with the person affected. There is general agreement that consideration of work organisation and job design, as well as the physical working environment, is essential to control RSI effectively (9).

NATIONAL STRATEGY
The response of the National Occupational Health and Safety Commission to the increasing problem with RSI was to establish a Committee to write a report and then develop a national strategy to implement the report. The National Strategy has six components:

1. Information
2. Standards
3. Research
4. Training
5. Statistics
6. Preventive Services

Conclusion

Reports of a decrease in reported cases of the condition are beginning to occur more frequently. Unfortunately, the lack of standardised reporting nationally prevents the presentation of a complete picture. However, the Australian Public Service has released figures which indicate a decline in some states (10).

In the March quarter 1986 there were 449 new cases of RSI reported. While the June quarter showed a drop to 354 new cases. A decrease was also reflected in figures which indicated staff years lost and numbers of persons involved in action related to the condition.

These figures are extremely encouraging for those of us involved in monitoring and evaluating the national strategy. Our actions to contain the situation have been undertaken with the view that problems which arise in the workplace must be met with solutions in the workplace and our strategy has been developed in consultation with labour and management and taking account of differences in individuals.

References

1. Australia, National Occupational Health and Safety Commission, Repetition Strain Injury A Report and Model Code of Practice, May 1986, AGPS, Canberra. para 5.42.
2. ibid. para 5.38
3. ibid. para 5.49
4. ibid. para 4.2
5. ibid. para 4.6
6. ibid. para 4.10
7. ibid. para 3.3
8. ibid. para 2.9
9. ibid. para 2.12
10. Australia, Public Service Board, Census of Repetition Strain Injury in the Australian Public Service, June Quarter; Public Service Board, Planning and Statistical Services Section, Canberra, 1986.

PREVENTION OF INJURIES RELATED TO PHYSICAL STRESS THROUGH
INTERVENTION BY LABOUR INSPECTORS

K. Kemmlert, Å. Nilsson, B. Andersson and
M. Bjurvald

National Board of Occupational Safety and Health,
171 84 Solna, Sweden

BACKGROUND

In Sweden a new law concerning workers' compensation took effect on the 1st of July, 1977. The changes in the law established a broader concept of the term "work injury" as well as increased monetary compensation.

On the first of January 1979 The National Board of Occupational Safety and Health (NBOSH) commenced a new system for collection of data concerning work injuries entitled the Information System on Occupational Injuries (ISA). The system is based on information concerning work injuries reported to ISA via the National Social Insurance Board.

The goal of ISA is to provide NBOSH with accurate information from which to develop preventative measures, both at the Research and Supervision Departments and at the Labour Inspectorate governed by the Board.

The Labour Inspectorate is divided into 19 districts where inspectors are responsible for a number of work places, making sure that legislation of the Board is complied with. The labour inspectors recieve a copy of every form reporting occupational injuries. Thus they are continuously provided with current information.

In 1983 the total number of reported cases of occupational injuries was 140 000. The cases consisted of accidents occuring in the work place, during transportation to or from work, and illnesses related to work.

The number of reported accidents in the work place was 105 729. Seventeen percent of these were the immediate result of stressful movements such as the manual handling of materials.

The number of reported illnesses due to work was 19 973. Of these 54% were related to the effect of overload e.g. sustained postures, manual materials handling or repetitive movements.

The transportation accidents numbered 14 298.

During the last few years the overall incidence of reported work injuries has decreased. In contrast, however, the number of stress related musculo-skeletal injuries has increased during the same period (NBOSH 1986).

It is well known that musculo-skeletal injuries result not only in financial loss to society and industry but also in personal suffering and restriction of activity.

When combined, accidents and illnesses due to work represent more than 20% of the total injuries reported. This percentage indicates the necessity of active prevention through the field of ergonomics.

A most valuable resource in the role of prevention is the Labour Inspectors. However ergonomic interventions constitute only 9% of the directives resulting from their inspections.

The prevention project

It is most likely that the injury forms would make a valuable basis for active prevention and provide effective help in questions of priority in supervision. In order to study the effects of more intense intervention in the field of ergonomics the Research and the Supervision Departments began a co-operative project with the Labour Inspectorate in the autumn of 1985.

Questions at issue:

The main questions in the project are as follows:

* Do the injury forms make an appropriate base for supervision in the field of ergonomics?

* Does a work place investigation on account of a reported injury give a more positive result than ordinary routines?

* Are there different backgrounds for occupational musculoskeletal injuries characterized as accidents compared to those characterized as illnesses?

PROCEDURE AND METHODS

The project started with a randomised collection of 200 cases of reported occupational injuries related to musculoskeletal stress. Fourteen inspectors, with different experience and background from three Inspectorate Districts, were invited to take part in the project. (All inspectors receive a brief training in ergonomics during their basic course, and most of them also have taken a one-week specialist course of ergonomics). For this project, they all participated in a two day course about ergonomic principles.

The education included the introduction of an observation method constructed at the Research Department (see form p. 7). This method is intended to simplify the work place assessments of occupational injuries. Thus the inspectors were trained, with the aid of photos and mock situations, to identify musculoskeletal stress factors which may have injurious effects.

The 200 reported cases were subdiveded into two groups of 100 reports each. One of these groups (studygroup) was investigated by the inspectors using the observation form. The other group (control group) was handled by routine.

After a year the study- and controlgroups are to be visited by the projectgroup, and changes in work station layout, work organization and attitudes of employers will be assessed.

Method of observation

The starting point for this method is a reported case of musculo-skeletal injury at a given work place. The form used to facilitate the analysis is designed as a flow chart, at the top of which is a horizontal row of pictures of the different body regions.

At the work place the investigation starts from the picture of the affected body region. The column below is followed vertically to white areas. These are connected with the far

Injury prevention and labour inspectors

right column, which presents a list (paragraphs 1-17) of physically stressful work factors.

This list of potential risk factors for musculo-skeletal stress on different body regions has been compiled from documentation in the available scientific documentation and agreements (see references 1-16). Most of this documentation has been published only in Swedish. A selection usually containing summaries in English is presented in the references. A list of the Swedish documentation can be obtained from the author. As regards the grey fields, such documentation has not been found.

After establishing if the work contains risk factors described in relevant questions 1-17, the investigator considers the factors a-f, which might cause additive injurious effects (see enclosed form   ).

Representative parts of the injured persons' work are to be investigated, i.e. parts of the work which are conducted for most of the time, or are look upon as particularly stressful to the musculo-skeletal system. Further investigation about other parts of the occupation should also be made to obtain information about all possible stress factors.

As a stressful task may give simultaneous symptoms in more than one region of the body, the load on regions other than the one of primary interest, may also have to be assessed.

The method may thus have to be repeated both for different parts of the work and for different body regions. It appears to be practical to use separate forms for different purposes.

Finally a concluding report is written, the wording of which could be collected from relevant points of the flow chart. As a matter of course, individual circumstances and other influencing factors not mentioned in the form should be added, as well as factors estimated to be of considerable influence in spite of their presence in a grey field.

Validity, reliability and utility

The validity and reliability of the method has recently been tested and the data are presently undergoing analysis for further presentation. Spontaneous reactions from the 30 investigators, who have used the method at repeated assess-

Method for the identification of musculo-skeletal stress factors which may have injurious effects.

Kemmlert, K. Kilbom, Å. (1986) National Board of Occupational Safety and Health, Research Department, Work Physiology Unit, 171 84 Solna, Sweden

Method of application.

- Find the injured body region
- Follow white fields to the right
- Do the work tasks contain any of the factors described?
- If so, tick where appropriate

Also take these factors into consideration:

a) the possibility to take breaks and pauses
b) the possibility to choose order and type of work tasks or pace of work
c) if the job is performed under time demands or psychological stress
d) if the work can have unusual or unexpected situations
e) presence of cold, heat, draught, noise or troublesome visual conditions
f) presence of jerks, shakes or vibrations

1. Is the walking surface uneven, sloping, slippery or nonresilient?
2. Is the space too limited for work movements or work materials?
3. Are tools and equipment unsuitably designed for the worker or the task?
4. Is the working height incorrectly adjusted?
5. Is the working chair poorly designed or incorrectly adjusted?
6. (If the work is performed whilst standing): Is there no possibility to sit and rest?
7. Is fatiguing (foot-pedal) work performed?
8. Is fatiguing leg work performed eg:
   a) repeated stepping up on stool, step etc.?
   b) repeated jumps, prolonged squatting or kneeling?
   c) one leg being used more often in supporting the body?
9. Is repeated or sustained work performed when the back is:
   a) flexed forward, more than 20°?
   b) severely flexed forward, more than 60°?
   c) bent sideways or twisted, more than 15°?
   d) severely twisted, more than 45°?
10. Is repeated or sustained work performed when the neck is:
    a) flexed forward, more than 15°?
    b) bent sideways or twisted, more than 15°?
    c) severely twisted, more than 45°?
    d) extended backwards?
11. Are loads lifted manually? Notice factors of importance as:
    a) periods of repetitive lifting
    b) weight of load
    c) awkward grasping of load
    d) awkward location of load at onset or end of lifting
    e) handling beyond forearm length
    f) handling below knee height
    g) handling above shoulder height
12. Is repeated, sustained or uncomfortable carrying, pushing or pulling of loads performed?
13. Is sustained work performed when one arm reaches forward or to the side without support?
14. Is there repetition of:
    a) similar work movements?
    b) similar work movements beyond comfortable reaching distance?
15. Is repeated or sustained manual work performed? Notice factors of importance as:
    a) weight of working materials or tools
    b) awkward grasping of working materials or tools
16. Are there high demands on visual capacity?
17. Is repeated work, with forearm and hand, performed with:
    a) twisting movements?
    b) forceful movements?
    c) uncomfortable hand positions?
    d) switches or keyboards?

ments, are that it helps them to concentrate on matters of importance and to put the findings into words.

The follow up study of the intervention effects is under way, and the conference report will give a broad out line of the project focusing on the observation method.

References

1. Bjurvald, M., Carlsöö, S., Hansson, J-E., och Sjöflot, L. Helkroppsvibrationer: en teknisk-fysiologisk studie av arbetsställningar och förarstolar (summary in English). Arbete och Hälsa 1973:7.

2. Chaffin, D. B., och Andersson, G. Occupational Biomechanics. John Wiley and Sons 1984.

3. Gamberale, F., Hansson, J-E., Jonsson, B., Kilbom, Å., och Ljungberg, A-S. Människans tolerans för lyft- och bärarbete (summary in English). Arbete och Hälsa 1981:16.

4. Hagberg, M. Occupational musculoskeletal stress and disorders of the neck and shoulder: a review of possible pathophysiology. Int Arch Occup Environ Health 53:269-78, 1984.

5. Harms-Ringdahl, K. On assessment of shoulder exercise and load-elicited pain in the cervical spine. Karolinska Institutet 1986.

6. Hunting, W., och Grandjean, E. Constrained postures in accounting machine operators. Applied Ergonomics 1980:11;145-9.

7. Kilbom, Å., Lagerlöf, E., Liew, M., och Broberg, E. An ergonomic study of notified cases of occupational musculo-skeletal disease. Proceedings of the International Conference on Occupational Ergonomics, Toronto 1984.

8. Kilbom, Å., Persson, J. and Jonsson, B. G. Disorders of the cervichobrachial region among female workers in the electronics industry. Int Journ of Ind Erg 1:37-47, 1986.

9. Kvarnström, S. Occurence of musculoskeletal disorders in a manufacturing industry with special attention to occupational shoulder disorders. Scan J Rehab Med, Suppl. 8:1-114, 1983.

10. Ljungberg, A-S., och Kilbom, Å. Lyftarbete och fysisk belastning hos sjukvårdspersonal inom långvården (summary in English). Arbete och Hälsa 1984:14.

11. NBOSH, Occupational Injuries 1983, National Board of Occupational Safety and Health, 1986.

12. NBOSH, Ergonoomic Injuries at work, Occupational Injuries 1984:37, National Board of Occupational Safety and Health, 1986

13. NIOSH, A Work Practices Guide for Manual Lifting, National Institute for Occupational Safety and Health, Tech. Report No 81-122, 1981.

14. Westgaard, R. H. and Aarås, A. Postural muscle strain as a causal factor in the developmet of musculo-skeletal illness. Applied Ergonomics 15.3, 162-74, 1984.

15. Wickström, G. Strain on the back in concrete reinforcement work. British Journal of Industrial Medicine 42:4;1985.

16. Winkel, J. En ergonomisk utvärdering av fotbesvär bland serveringspersonal. Högskolan i Luleå (summary in English). TULEA 1982:26.

REPETITIVE STRAIN INJURIES AMONG SERVICE PERSONNEL ON NORTH
SEA OIL PLATFORMS

M. Wærsted and R.H. Westgaard
Institute of Work Physiology, Gydas vei 8, Oslo 3, Norway

INTRODUCTION
Catering personnel on the Statfjord oil field have a 12 hour working day for 14 days, followed by 21 days at home. The work tasks are varied, involving mainly catering and cleaning functions, but time constraints ensure that work is carried out at considerable pace for long periods of time. There are also clear differences in work tasks between various subgroups of workers, such as cooks and service workers, resulting in different patterns of work strain. High sick leave among the catering personnel caused considerable concern, and was one of the incentives behind the initiation of a research program in 1983. The program included documentation of ergonomic and psycho-social aspects of the catering work, as well as documentation of health situation and work load for the catering personnel. This paper presents results from the analysis of sick leave and musculo-skeletal complaints. A project-report (in norwegian) mainly addressed to employers and employees is published (Westgaard et al., 1987).

METHODS
Two methods were used for quantification of musculo-skeletal injuries: Analysis of sick leave (including information on medical diagnosis) of catering personnel employed on the platforms of the Statfjord oil-field in the years 1978-1983. The analysis is based on 1350 sick leaves over 1600 man-labour years, by 299 female and 311 male workers. Further details of the epidemiological procedure are described by Westgaard & al. (1986). The second method is based on analysis of responses to a questionnaire regarding symptoms of musculo-skeletal injuries presented to workers in the autumn of 1983. The questionnaire was

handed out to 284 workers, and was returned by 198 (69%).

RESULTS AND DISCUSSION

Fig.1 shows days lost through sick leave due to musculo-skeletal injuries at different body locations, as a percentage of possible work time for different categories of catering personnel. Female service workers record the highest rate of musculo-skeletal sick leave at 4.4% of possible work time, accounting for about 40% of all sick leave for this group of workers. Female cooks record a similar rate of musculo-skeletal injuries, but the statistics for this group is inflated due to a single leg injury of 8 months duration (1.3% of possible work time for this group).

The high rate of musculo-skeletal injuries for female service workers relative to other groups of catering personnel is mainly due to higher rate of injuries in neck, shoulders and arms. This difference in occurrence of shoulder, neck, arm injuries (2.5% sick leave for female service workers vs. 0.3 to 1.0% for other groups) is likely to be caused by conditions at work. The occurrence of such injuries among female service workers has been shown to increase with time of employment, that is time of exposure to load (fig.6 of Westgaard & al., 1986). Furthermore, 65 percent of female service workers feel that symptoms of such injuries (i.e. pain or discomfort located to the appropriate body structures) are developing as a consequence of physical work strain while performing their work duties.

Additional evidence of an association between work strain and the development of musculo-skeletal injuries is provided by Fig.2 which shows fraction of workers reporting discomfort or pain at any body location (Fig.2A), in neck, shoulders (Fig.2B) or in legs, feet (Fig.2C) at different days of their off-shore duty period. Results from two subgroups of female service workers are shown: cabin workers who perform cleaning tasks under considerable time constraint throughout their duty period, and mess workers who have a more varied work pattern (bringing supplies, filling drink dispensers, clearing tables, washing dishes etc.), but with a general requirement of performing most of their work tasks standing up or walking. It is seen that symptoms of pain or discomfort are accumulating over the 14-day duty period to about the same extent for both groups (Fig.2A). However, there is a differential effect when local body structures are considered: cabin workers show a marked increase in the incidence of symptoms in shoulders and neck over the off-shore duty period, while a similar

Figure 1. Percent sick leave due to musculo-skeletal injuries (days ill of possible work time) in the years 1978-1983 for six different categories of catering personnel on the Statfjord oil-field. Shoulder-neck-arm (dark), low back (double hatching) and other (single hatching) musculo-skeletal injuries are shown. The analysis is based on the following number of man-labour years: female service workers 687 years, male service workers 382 years, female cooks 51 years, male cooks 279 years, male bakers 61 years and male supervisors 98 years.

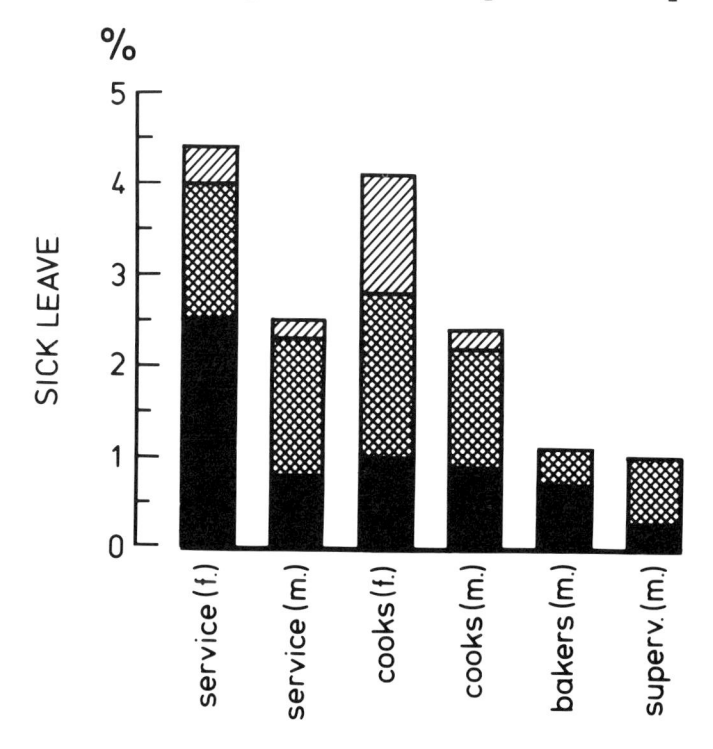

effect is seen for mess workers in legs and feet. Symptoms in low back and lower arms were occurring at a similar and lower rate for the two groups, the incidence of symptoms in lower arms increasing from 0 to 20% over the duty period.

The results of Fig.2 are consistent with the hypothesis that the development of symptoms of musculo-skeletal illness is a consequence of continuous work strain in local body structures. In particular, the results support the hypothesis that musculo-skeletal injuries in shoulders, neck and arms develop as a consequence of continuous work strain while performing cleaning tasks.

156   Musculoskeletal disorders at work

Figure 2. Fraction of persons in two subgroups of female service workers (cabin work, 30 subjects; mess work, 20 subjects) who report complaints at different times of their off-shore duty period. A. Complaints regardless of body location. B. Complaints in shoulders, neck. C. Complaints in legs, feet.

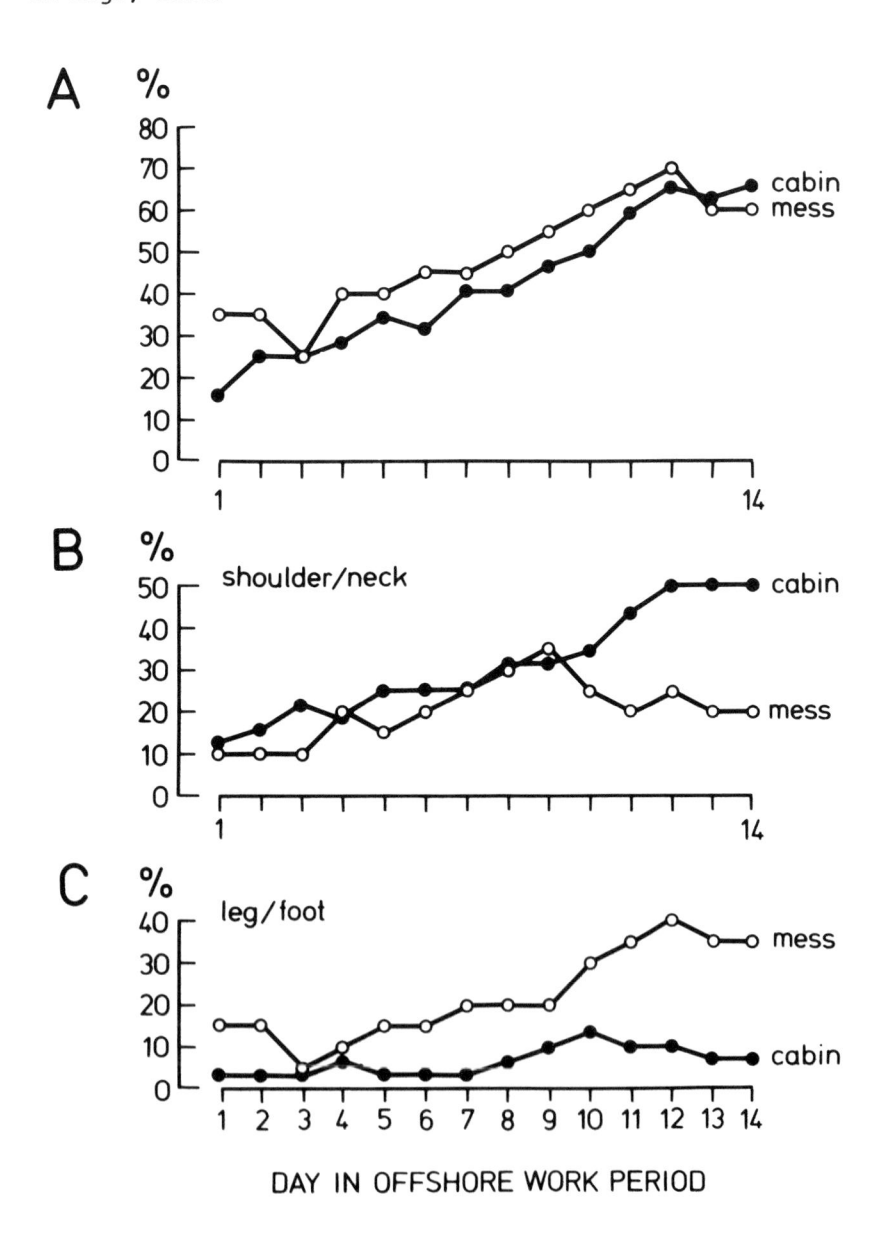

DAY IN OFFSHORE WORK PERIOD

Load on the trapezius muscles as well as flexor and extensor muscles in the lower arms was measured by electromyographic recordings. Results of recordings from the trapezius muscles while performing cabin duties are documented elsewhere (figs. 3 and 5, Westgaard & al., 1986). The load pattern was intermittent with a low static component (about 1% MVC, as defined by Jonsson, 1978), but with no pauses of more than a few seconds appearing while working. Work was carried out for about 8 hours during the 12 hour working day, with periods of continuous work lasting as long as 2 hours. Muscle load while performing other work tasks is less well documented, but available recordings suggest that the load pattern for a variety of tasks is similar to that seen for cabin work. A possible difference is the appearance of longer breaks, from 10 seconds to several minutes, in the trapezius load pattern. These breaks may either appear as an unloading of a muscle while other muscles continue working, or as a result of spontaneous pauses in the work pattern.

The differential rate of injuries among subgroups of female service workers in terms of development of shoulder, neck injuries is not known. Also, a service worker may perform mess duties one off-shore period and cabin duties the next. However, the results of Fig.2 may be interpreted as evidence for an increased risk of developing shoulder, neck injuries among cabin workers relative to mess workers. This together with the results of the load measurements suggest that a further reduction in intensity of trapezius load is likely to be less effective than an increase in number of pauses of at least 10-20 seconds duration in the load pattern, for reducing the risk of developing a shoulder, neck injury.

The load pattern for muscles in the forearm is very similar to those recorded for the trapezius muscle, both with regard to time pattern and intensity. The rate of injuries in lower arms among female service workers is about 50% of that recorded for the shoulder, neck region, but is much higher than for low arm injuries among other groups of service workers. It can be argued, in a similar way as for shoulder, neck injuries, that work strain in the lower arm is a major cause of these injuries and that the load on these muscles is excessive. It is then of interest to note that injuries in the lower arms happen at a much lower rate than shoulder, neck injuries despite similar load on trapezius and low arm muscles. Also, injuries of muscles in the forearm appear to affect the muscle tendons (common diagnoses are tendinitis, tenosynovitis, peritendinitis, epicondylitis) to a much larger extent than for the shoulder muscles. This suggests a differential sensitivity of different muscles to the same load pattern in terms of development of injuries, and also that different substructures of the muscle organ may be a limiting factor for different muscles.

Male and female service workers and cooks developed injuries in the low back to about the same extent (1.3 to 1.8% sick leave), while bakers recorded a much lower rate of low back injuries (0.4%). This is again consistent with the observed work pattern where service workers and cooks of both sexes perform frequent lifting tasks, to a much larger extent than bakers. Supervisors (0.7% sick leave due to back injuries) perform heavy lifting operations twice a week when receiving food supplies from service vessels. Low back load is therefore also likely to exceed an acceptable limit for some groups of catering workers, but it is not possible to elaborate on this observation as there was no quantitative evaluation of low back load.

CONCLUSION

The results of this study emphasize the need for short rest pauses in an otherwise continuous work pattern. It is also unlikely that an acceptable level of load on specific muscles can be defined only in terms of load intensity, without specifying time constraints for maintaining this load.

REFERENCES

Jonsson, B., 1978, Kinesiology – with special reference to electromyographic kinesiology. In Contemporary Clinical Neurophysiology, EEG Suppl. No. 34, edited by W.A. Cobb & H. Van Duijn (Elsevier, Amsterdam), pp. 417-428.

Westgaard, R.H., Wærsted, M., Jansen, T. & Aarås, A., 1986, Muscle load and illness associated with constrained body postures. In The Ergonomics of Working Postures, edited by N. Corlett, J. Wilson & I. Manenica, (Taylor & Francis, London), pp. 3-18.

Westgaard, R.H. et.al., 1987, Arbeidsmiljø, belastningslidelser og sykefravær blant forpleiningspersonell på Statfjordfeltet, (Universitetsforlaget, Bergen).

TRAINING IN SAFE LIFTING:

ARE THE METHODS TAUGHT USED BY WORKERS?

ST-VINCENT, M., LORTIE, M., TELLIER, C.

INSTITUT DE RECHERCHE EN SANTÉ ET SÉCURITÉ
DU TRAVAIL DU QUÉBEC
Safety and Ergonomics Research Program
505 de Maisonneuve Blvd. W., Montreal, Quebec, H3A 3C2

INTRODUCTION

Recent studies have suggested that training in safe lifting is ineffective in preventing occupational low back pain (Snook et al, 1978; Dehlin et al, 1981; Stubbs et al, 1983). However, it is actually not known whether it is ineffective because previously taught methods are not used or because these methods are intrinsically ineffective. The present study was designed to assess the first hypothesis in hospital workers since they are particularly exposed to low back pain. A field study was conducted in a geriatric hospital, and handling methods used by workers were compared to those taught during training. Two specific objectives were set: (1) to determine whether the methods taught are used or not, and (2) in the latter case, to characterize and explain the main deviations from these methods.

METHODS

The observational procedure: The handling methods used in the workplace have been characterized using an observational procedure designed specifically to describe patient handling operations (St-Vincent et al, 1985). This procedure allows taught methods to be described as well as more varied ones which can be observed in the workplace. The handling method is characterized both as a function of the static component (holds and posture at the beginning of the lifting) and of the dynamic component of handling. The posture at the start is defined as a function of the position of the feet (angle, distance apart), the amount the knees are bent (straight, somewhat bent, or very bent) and of the back posture in the sagittal plane (straight, somewhat bent, or very bent: > 45°). The dynamic component is described as a function of three major factors: 1) direction of the effort applied (vertical: lifting, lowering; horizontal: pushing, pulling, shoulder axis direction), 2) back movements during the effort (∧ sagittal, lateral bending, twisting), 3) motor component involved (arms, back, legs, type of leg movement: vertical, lateral or antero-posterior weight transfer). This last parameter essentially documents the dynamic contribution of the different body structures and does not take into account the static work which can be carried out. This observational procedure was validated using a video tape recording showing 44 handling tasks. This recording was seen twice by each of two observers who were to carry out the field study. The intra- and inter-observer reproducibility, evaluated for all the observational criteria, are respectively 93% ± 5% and 91% ± 7% (mean ± standard deviation).

The field study: This observational procedure was used during a field study carried out by two observers in a geriatric hospital. Four units were selected, and 33 trained orderlies were observed while they worked. A total of 1,400 handling operations were described. These operations were divided into 5 major categories **(Table I)**

TABLE 1. DEFINITION AND DISTRIBUTION OF THE OBSERVED HANDLING OPERATIONS.

Code of the operation	Definition	N	%
	IN-PLACE HANDLING OPERATION	346	25%
OP1	Moving a patient up in the bed	144	10%
OP2	Sitting a patient on the edge of the bed (patient who had been lying)	140	10%
OP3	Laying a patient down who had been sitting on the edge of the bed	62	5%
TR OPER	TRANSFER OPERATION	1000	71%
OP4	-- TAKING --	500	35%
OP4A	From bed	226	16%
OP4b	From chair	274	19%
OP5	-- PUTTING DOWN --	500	35%
OP5A	On bed	162	11%
OP5B	In chair	338	25%
	OTHER OPERATIONS	54	4%
TOTAL		1 400	100%

3 are in-place handling operations carried out in the bed, whereas the 2 others correspond to taking up and putting down operations observed during transfers. In Table 1, the latter two operations were divided into 2 sub-groups depending on whether the operation was carried out from the bed or from the chair. Six other types of operations which were observed in a much more marginal way, were grouped in the category "other".

The training program and its evaluation: The training given is based mainly on the teaching of general principles to be applied to various handling tasks. To assess whether this training was applied, we determined the frequency of use of the six major principles which are taught: 1) working with the knees extremely bent, 2) the feet far apart, 3) pointed in the direction of the movement, 4) with the back straight, 5) during the effort, with the back posture constant, and 6) carrying out the movement using the lower limbs exclusively. It is also recommended that horizontal efforts be used when possible, in order to minimize efforts which are strictly vertical. The influence of the handling operation on the use of these principles was also evaluated.

RESULTS

For all of the handling operations described, the work profile taught was hardly ever used; in fact, the simultaneous application of the 6 principles taught was seen in only 1% of the cases. As Table II shows, the

TABLE II. FREQUENCY THAT TAUGHT PRINCIPLES ARE USED AND FREQUENCY OF OBSERVED DEVIATIONS.

HANDLING PRINCIPLE	RECOMMENDED CONDITION	OBSERVED CONDITION		
1:Feet:parallel or at angle	With angle 16%	Parallel 84%		
2:Feet:close or apart	Far apart 25%	Somewhat apart 69%	Close 6%	
3:Knee bending	Extremely bent 11%	Somewhat bent 24%	Straight 65%	
4:Back sagittal bending	Straight back 18%	Somewhat bent 61%	Very bent 21%	
5:Back motion	Constant posture 11%	Sagitt. 78%	Lateral bending 36%	Twisting 15%
6:Motor struct.	Legs 33%	Back 89%	Arms 96%	

frequency of use of each of the principles taken separately is also not very significant. In a majority of cases, contrary to what is taught, handling is carried out with the legs straight, the feet parallel and close together, with the back somewhat bent; during the effort the back moves (most often it is moved in the sagittal plane, but as we shall see, lateral bending and twisting are concentrated in certain categories of operations) and the handling is carried out using the arms and the back. In addition, it is very rare that strictly horizontal efforts are used (as recommended): 98% of the in-place handling operations and 65% of the transfer operations are carried out with efforts having both a vertical and horizontal component whereas 45% of the transfer operations are carried out using strictly vertical efforts. The principle which is most often applied is the use of the legs, observed however in only 33% of the cases. Contrary also to what was taught, the legs are very rarely used by themselves; in 81% of the cases they are used together with the back and the arms.

Table III shows that the deviations observed with respect to use of the back and the legs vary according to the type of operation carried out. All three in-place handling

TABLE III. EFFECT OF THE HANDLING OPERATION ON THE USE OF THE BACK AND THE LEGS. For each of the 6 described parameters, the effect of the operation was evaluated by a χ^2 test;**the differences are significant (P <.001).

		Total %	TRANSFER				IN-PLACE HANDLING		
			CHAIR		BED				
			OP4b (Tak.)	OP5b (Put)	OP4A (Tak.)	OP5A (Put)	OP1	OP2	OP3
Use of back	**	89%	92%	87%	92%	96%	71%	98%	98%
Use of legs	**	33%	57%	42%	24%	17%	16%	24%	15%
Lateral bending	**	26%	21%	22%	26%	43%	64%	78%	66%
Twisting	**	15%	13%	14%	24%	40%	0%	1%	3%
Δ sagittal	**	87%	88%	83%	83%	85%	10%	96%	98%
Deep sag bending	**	21%	26%	12%	15%	9%	0%	53%	36%

operations are characterized by very little use of the
legs and a marked presence of lateral bending. The operations of "sitting edge of bed (OP2)" (and to a lesser
degree the operations of "laying down in bed (OP3)") are
also characterized by a high frequency of extreme forward
bending. Transfer operations carried out in the bed,
especially putting down operations, present similar tendencies (little use of the legs, marked presence of lateral bending) and in addition are characterized by a rather
high frequency of twisting. On the other hand, transfer
operations to the chair are distinguished by more frequent
use of the legs and a marked absence of both twisting and
lateral bending. The use of the back and movements in the
sagittal plane are characteristics common to all operations, with the exception of the "moving up in the bed
(OP1)" operations where displacement in the sagittal plane
is almost nonexistant.

DISCUSSION AND CONCLUSION

The results presented show very clearly that in the hospital visited, the training is hardly applied at all and
that the observed deviations are a function of the operations carried out. There is no operation where all of the
taught principles are used because in most of the cases
the back is the motor component. If, however, the non-use
of legs and the marked presence of lateral bending or
twisting are retained as points of major deviation, it is
possible to distinguish two main types of handling. The
first type corresponds to handling operations carried out
at the bed. In this type of handling operation, whether
it be handling-in-place or transfer operations, training
is hardly applied; the legs are hardly used and there is a
high presence of lateral bending or twisting (twisting are
restricted mainly to the putting down operations carried
at the bed). On the other hand, in handling operations
carried out at the chair training is more often applied:
the legs are frequently used and twisting and lateral
bending are less frequent. These results suggest that
actual training is hardly adapted to handling operations
carried out at the bed particularly to the in-place
handling operations which are the most often carried out
with efforts having a horizontal component. In fact, the
principles which are taught are based essentially on the
laboratory study of symmetrical lifting operations carried
out in the sagittal plane. It is possible that the principles which are true for this type of handling cannot

be transposed integrally to handling operations which are not vertical and are asymmetric. These handling operations, especially those carried out at the bed, undoubtedly impose postural constraints which are not present in sagittal handling operations. One could also wonder about the validity of using the legs during horizontal handling operations. In most of the training programs, it is in fact recommended that these handling operations be carried out using weight transfer. In the program evaluated, for example, a patient is to be moved to the head of the bed by sliding him while using a lateral weight transfer as the only driving force. It is doubtful that this transfer of weight can by itself generate sufficient force to carry out the displacement, particularly when forces of friction are involved. The mechanical efficiency of such weight transfers has in any case never been demonstrated in the laboratory. The fact that they are so infrequently used suggests that they are not really advantageous.

In conclusion, this study shows that actual training programs are not an effective prevention strategy because the methods which are taught are rarely used. A better understanding of the constraints encountered during patient handling would be necessary to plan a more realistic prevention strategy.

REFERENCES

Dehlin O., Berg S., Andersson G.B., Grimby G., 1981. Effect of physical training and ergonomic counselling on the psychological perception of work and on the subjective assessment of low-back insufficiency. Scandinavian Journal of Rehabilitation Medicine, 13, 1-9.

St-Vincent M., Lortie M., Tellier C., 1985. Les programmes de formation dans le secteur hospitalier, leur évaluation par l'étude des comportements de travail. Proceedings of the Annual Conference of the Human Factors Association of Canada (19e), 59-62.

Snook S.H., Campanelli R.A., Hart J.WW., 1978. A study of three preventive approaches to low back injury. Journal of Occupational Medecine, 20(7), 478-481.

Stubbs A.A., Buckle P.W., Hudson M.P., Rivers P.M., 1983. Back pain in the nursing profession II. The effectiveness of training. Ergonomics, 26(8), 767-779.

TESTS OF MANUAL WORKING CAPACITY
AND THE PREDICTION OF LOW BACK PAIN

J.D.G. Troup, T.K. Foreman, C.E. Baxter and D. Brown

Department of Orthopædic and Accident Surgery
University of Liverpool
P.O. Box 147
Liverpool   L69 3BX

The aim of this survey, commissioned by the Health and Safety Executive, was to test the hypothesis that tests of manual working capacity, suitable for use by occupational health staff, would serve to identify those individuals who were susceptible to low back pain (LBP).

The subject-material was 2,891 volunteers who were questioned about their experience of LBP and given a battery of tests. One year later they were sent a postal questionnaire to which 88.7% responded.

The best predictor was a previous history of LBP; but its predictive value was enhanced by the test-results. None of the tests, or combination of tests, served reliably to identify new cases of LBP.

INTRODUCTION

Pre-employment health screening has been suggested as an approach to the prevention of LBP but there has been no evidence that it will serve to identify those who are susceptible to their first attacks. Previous experience of LBP is the best predictor (Troup & Edwards 1985).

Isometric strength testing was found to be a predictor in army recruits (Karvonen et al. 1980) and Biering-Sörensen (1984) reported an endurance test of back muscle strength to be predictive in volunteers in a health survey. In an industrial environment, isometric strength testing in relation to the forces required at work was found to have predictive value (Chaffin et al. 1978; Keyserling et al. 1980a, b) but others have found that LBP can be precipitated by such testing (Hansson et al.1984). Reductions in dynamic trunk flexor strength (incapacity to perform a 'sit-up') and of lumbar sagittal mobility are more evident in those with previous LBP (Troup et al. 1981). In addition, Snook (1978) reported that LBP at work was commoner whenever the loads handled at work exceeded his tabulated values for acceptable maxima. However, his data were obtained using experienced industrial workers after one week of training and his methods were not designed as a routine screening test.

Two new psychophysical tests of lifting strength were developed: a dynamic lifting test, the Rating of Acceptable Load (RAL), by Griffin et al. (1984), who showed that RALs were less in those with LBP; and a test of acceptable isometric lifting force (AILF) (Foreman et al. 1984, Baxter et al. 1985). These tests, together with maximal isometric lifting strength (MlLS), tests of lumbar mobility and of respiratory function, the 'sit-up' and a number of anthropometric tests were administered on admission to the prospective survey.

METHODS
Subject-Material

Volunteers were recruited from University, Technical College, Hospital, Ambulance and Fire Service employees. A total of 2,891 (1,150 females and 1,741 males) were questioned about previous LBP and tested. All were tested at or near their work places under conditions that would be applicable to pre-employment health screening. Twelve months later they received postal questionnaires on subsequent LBP to which 2,564 (88.7%) responded.

LBP Questionnaires

Subjects who reported previous LBP were asked if they experienced it daily, weekly, monthly, a few times a year, less than once a year or if they had no further episodes. They were asked to identify the first, worst and most recent attacks of LBP, for how long they were away from work and the intensity of LBP on each of the occasions using a 21-point scale.

On postal follow-up they were asked, in addition, about absence from work, injuries and problems with manual handling.

The Test-Battery
The following tests were administered:
- body weight
- body height
- height at C7

- iliac crest height
- anterior superior iliac spine distance (ASIS)
- chest circumference
- lumbar flexed curve angle (FLEX)
- lumbar extended curve angle (EXT)
- dynamic trunk flexion ('SIT-UP' test)
- acceptable isometric lifting force at knee and waist level ($AILF_k$ and $AILF_w$)
- maximal isometric lifting strength at knee and waist level ($MILS_k$ and $MILS_w$)
- rating of acceptable load (RAL)
- weight handling skill (total pursuit rotor time on target)(PRT)
- respiratory function tests (FEVC, $FEV_{0.5}$, $FEV_{1.0}$, PEF, FIVC, $FIV_{0.5}$, $FIV_{1.0}$, PIF).

Storage and Analysis of Data

All analyses were made using SPSSX, employing the following statistical methods:- descriptive statistics; analysis of variance by 'ONEWAY'; multiple range testing to identify differences between groups; chi-square tests; and discriminant analysis. Data were corrected for age by deriving regression equations based on three variables - pain-group, age and sex - and their three interactions.

RESULTS

Previous LBP

No previous back pain ('non-backs') was reported by 39.6% of females and 39.6% of males, their mean ages being 31.1 (±10.5) and 33.7 (±9.9) years respectively. Back pain was experienced not more than once monthly ('mild backs') by 42.0% of females and 48.1% of males (chi-squ. =10.25, p<0.001): their mean ages respectively being 35.5 (±12.1) and 36.9 (±10.5) years. Back pain at least once a week ('chronic backs') was reported by 18.4% females and 12.2% of males (chi-squ.=20.52, p<0.001) whose ages averaged 39.2 (±12.3) and 40.3 (±11.2) years respectively. Thus, more females tended to experience chronic LBP than males; more males experienced mild back pain than females; while the 'chronic backs' of both sexes were significantly older.

LBP at the time of testing was reported by 16.3% of females and 14.2% of males. While 9.7% of females and 6.5% of males experienced LBP for the first time during the preceding twelve months. Sickness-absence was longest and pain intensity rated highest for the worst attack.

Both absence and pain intensity were less in the most recent episode, sickness-absence and pain intensity being closely related (p<0.001).

LBP and Test-Data
Females with LBP were heavier and had larger chest circumferences but other anthropometric variables were poorly related to pain-group.
Lumbar EXT and the capacity to SIT-UP were both reduced in those with LBP. Of the tests of lifting strength, RAL, $AILF_K$, and $MILS_k$ were all reduced in the 'chronic backs' compared with 'non-backs' (p<0.001) in both sexes. Of the respiratory function tests, $FEV_{0.5}$ and $FEV_{1.0}$ were less in those with LBP while PIF was higher.
When the data were age-corrected, the greatest difference between pain-groups for males and females was for $AILF_k$: the 'chronic/non' ratios being 84% and 68% respectively. Although the differences between pain-groups were less for the respiratory function tests than for EXT, RAL, AILF and MILS, the goodness of fit was higher, particularly for PEF.

Follow-Up Data
The relation between original and follow-up pain-groups was as follows:

original	sex	n=	non-backs	follow-up mild backs	'chronics'
non-backs	m	622	496 (79.7%)	87 (14.0%)	39 (6.3%)
	f	392	298 (76.0%)	57 (14.5%)	37 (9.4%)
mild backs	m	736	343 (46.6%)	265 (36.0%)	128 (17.4%)
	f	407	170 (41.8%)	116 (28.5%)	121 (29.7%)
'chronics'	m	188	12 (6.4%)	20 (10.6%)	156 (83.0%)
	f	184	19 (10.3%)	13 (7.1%)	152 (82.6%)
		2,529	1,338 (52.9%)	558 (22.1%)	633 (25.0%)

Thus, about 80% of the original 'chronics' remained in the same category on follow-up and, likewise, just under 80% of the 'non-backs' remained free of LBP. Altogether, 59.3% of the population continued in the same pain-group. On follow-up, 19% reported an injury and 14% a manual handling problem, particularly nurses and ambulance staff.

Test-Data and LBP-Prediction
From the original and follow-up pain-groups, five LBP-groups were defined:-

                        'non' to 'non'
                        'non' to 'new'
                        'mild' to 'mild'
                        'mild' to 'chronic'
                       'chronic' to 'chronic'.
Discriminant analysis was undertaken to compare predicted
LBP-groups with actual LBP-groups on follow-up. Using 8
variables (EXT, SIT-UP, RANGE, AGE, RAL, $AILF_K$, $MILS_K$
and $AILF_W$) predictions of LBP were as follows:

		predicted group (males)				
actual group	n=	1	2	3	4	5
1: non-non	486	460	0	13	0	13
2: non-new	125	116	0	7	0	2
3: mild-mild	260	219	0	23	0	18
4: mild-chron	124	100	0	14	0	10
5: chron-chron	121	82	0	16	0	23

		predicted group (females)				
actual group	n=	1	2	3	4	5
1: non-non	288	264	2	3	6	13
2: non-new	92	78	1	2	4	7
3: mild-mild	114	85	1	6	8	14
4: mild-chron	119	75	2	2	8	32
5: chron-chron	110	50	0	2	5	53

Thus only 19% of male and 48% of female 'chronic-chronics'
were predicted and the overall accuracy of prediction for
the five pain-groups was 45% for males and 46% for females.
    A ninth variable was then added, 'LBPfreq', using the
answers to the original questionnaire from '1'= 'pain
experienced daily' to '7'= 'no pain', to give the following
predictions:

		predicted group (males)				
actual group	n=	1	2	3	4	5
1: non-non	486	486	0	0	0	0
2: non-new	125	125	0	0	0	0
3: mild-mild	260	58	0	187	15	0
4: mild-chron	124	23	0	85	16	0
5: chron-chron	121	0	0	0	0	121

The overall accuracy for the males was 72.6% with 100%
prediction of both 'non-non' and 'chronic-chronic'
LBP-groups. For females, the overall accuracy of
prediction was 70.8% with only two errors in the prediction
of 'non-non' and 'chronic-chronic' LBP-groups:-

		predicted group (females)				
actual group	n=	1	2	3	4	5
1: non-non	288	286	2	0	0	0
2: non-new	92	90	2	0	0	0
3: mild-mild	114	18	0	37	59	0
4: mild-chron	119	15	0	27	77	0
5: chron-chron	110	0	0	0	0	110

In 437 males and 239 females who had replied to additional questions on smoking and coughing, there was a significant relation between chest symptoms and LBP but none between LBP and smoking. Using LBPfreq, WEIGHT, CHEST CIRC., AGE and the 8 RESPIRATORY FUNCTION tests, the five LBP-groups were predicted with an overall accuracy of 72.9% in males and 79.9% in females, and 100% of 'non-non' and 'chronic-chronic' groups.

REFERENCES

Baxter, C.E., Foreman, T.K. & Troup, J.D.G. 1985, In Oborne, D. (Ed.), Contemporary Ergonomics 1985, (London: Taylor & Francis Ltd), p.222.
Biering-Sörensen, F. 1984, Spine, 9, 106.
Chaffin, D.B., Herrin, G.D. & Keyserling, W.M. 1978, Journal of Occupational Medicine, 20, 403.
Foreman, T.K., Baxter, C.E. & Troup, J.D.G. 1984, Ergonomics, 27, 1283.
Griffin, A.B., Troup, J.D.G. & Lloyd, D.C.E.F. 1984, Ergonomics, 27, 305.
Hansson, T.H., Bigos, S.J., Wortley, M.K. & Spengler, D.M. 1984, Spine, 9, 720.
Karvonen, M.J., Viitasalo, J.T., Komi, P.V., Nummi, J. & Järvinen, T. 1980, Scandinavian Journal of Rehabilitation Medicine, 12, 53.
Keyserling, W.M., Herrin, G.D. & Chaffin, D.B. 1980a, Journal of Occupational Medicine, 22, 332.
Keyserling, W.M., Herrin, G.D., Chaffin, D.B., Armstrong, T. & Foss, M.L. 1980b, American Industrial Hygiene Association Journal, 41, 730.
Snook, S.H. 1978, Ergonomics, 21, 963.
Troup, J.D.G. & Edwards, F.C. 1985, Manual Handling and Lifting: An Information and Literature Review with Special Reference to the Back, Health and Safety Executive, London: HMSO.
Troup, J.D.G., Martin. J.W. & Lloyd, D.C.E.F. 1981, Spine, 6, 61.

THREE DIMENSIONAL NON-INVASIVE ASSESSMENT OF LUMBAR BRACE IMMOBILIZATION OF THE SPINE

Dorsky, S.; Buchalter, D.; Kahanovitz, N.; Nordin, M.

Hospital for Joint Diseases Orthopaedic Instititue.
301 East 17th Street,
New York, New York 10003 USA

The use of braces is one of the most common modalities of treatment utilized for various pathologies relating to the spine. Orthopedists, physiatrists, and many primary care physicians all routinely prescribe braces for the treatment of back ailments. Back braces can be classified as either corrective or supportive types of braces. The corrective brace is usually utilized as an active form of correction for a spinal deformity such as scoliosis or kyphosis. The supportive type of brace works by means of a passive mechanism and can be either soft or rigid. Braces are routinely used for a variety of diagnoses including low back sprain or strain, spondylolisthesis, or support for the post-surgical patient.

Perry (1970) surveyed 150 orthopedists to evaluate their prescribing patterns for back braces. It was noted that the clinical indications for the use of a brace were quite clear; however, there was no clear consensus concerning the type of support that should be used for a particular diagnosis. Practitioners when treating the same condition will often prescribe different braces, or at times even alternately use two or more types of braces in treating the same problem (Morris 1974, Norton 1957). Part of this problem exists due to a lack of sufficient information as to what a brace actually does for the patient.

The purpose of this study was to determine the restriction of motion in three planes as well as the perceived comfort provided by four

commonly prescribed lumbar braces.
Materials and Methods
The measurement of motion in the spine was made utilizing the 3 - Space Analyzer (McDonnel Douglass Electronics Company Colchester, Vermont, 05446 U.S.A.) (Three Space Tracher 1985). The concept of measuring spine motion with this device resulted as an outgrowth of work done by McDonnell Douglass for the aerospace industry. The device provides a non-invasive technique for determining motion.

A low frequency magnetic field is generated and multiple sensors are used to determine the orientation of each sensor in a magnetic field. The total sampling rate of the equipment is 60 sets of data per second which can be divided evenly up to four sensors. The data is collected and analyzed providing the basis for calculating the motion between any two sensors. It is possible to account simultaneously for motion in three planes.

Figure 1 shows the 3-Space Analyzer with sensors and the transmitting antennor source of the magnetic field. This method has been previously tested for normal range of motion and has proven to be both accurate and reproducible (Dorsky et al 1986). The results were compared to data obtained by other methods and were highly comparable (Hanley et al 1976, Macrae & Wright 1969, Moll & Wright 1969, Portck 1983).

Figure 1 shows the 3-Space Tracker with the sensors and source in the far right corner of the table.

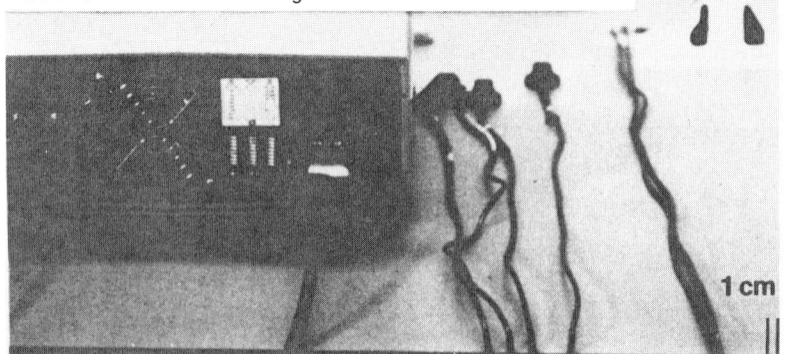

In this study, 33 healthy subjects ranging in age from 16 to 41 years were tested. The braces included the Raney jacket, the Camp lace-up corset, a molded-polypropylene thoraco-lumbar-sacral orthosis (TLSO) and a common elastic corset (Figures 2-5).

Each subject was initially placed in an upright relaxed, posture before performing free motion in three planes, with the sagittal plane representing flexion and extension, the coronal plane representing lateral bending, and the transverse plane representing rotation.

The braces were fitted by a trained orthotist. Each subject acted as his/her own control making it possible to calculate the percent reduction in motion provided by each brace.

Figure 2 shows the Raney jacket.

Figure 3 shows the Camp corset.

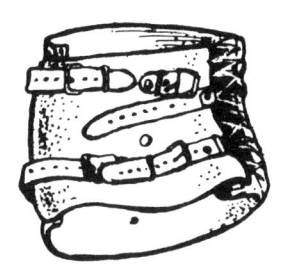

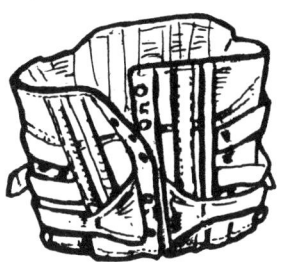

Figure 4 shows the molded TLSO.

Figure 5 shows the elastic corset.

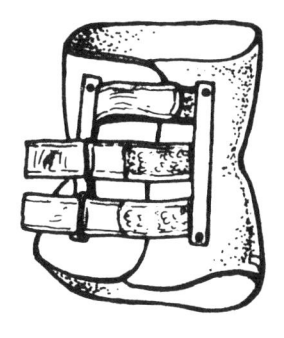

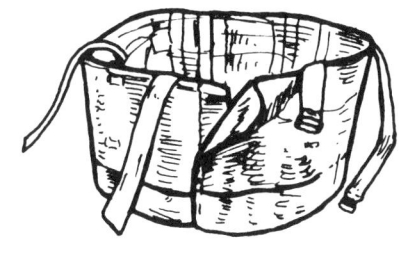

After testing for the maximal range of motion in all three planes, each subject was randomly fitted with each of the four braces. The sensors were placed on standard anatomic landmarks at C7, T12 and the sacrum enabling the measurements of motion across both the thoracic and lumbar spine. All testing was performed by the same individuals to provide consistency in the testing protocol.

All subjects were asked to rate the comfort of each brace on a 1 to 10 scale as originally described by Chapman et al (1985). A scale of 10 denoted complete freedom of movement with no restriction and comfort approaching not wearing a brace. A score of 1 denoted intolerable restriction and discomfort to the subject.

Results

The measured unrestricted motion in the lumbar spine revealed mean values of 70° of flexion/extension, 31° of lateral bending and 8° rotation. The greatest restriction of flexion and extension was found in the Raney Jacket with 79% restriction, followed closely by the molded TLSO with 69% restriction. The Camp corset provided 53% restriction where the elastic corset provided only 31% restriction. A much greater degree of overall restriction was found in lateral bending where the molded TLSO provided the most restriction with 94% reduction. All braces provided greater than 60% restriction of lateral bending. The restriction in rotation was inconsequential due to the limited rotation which exists under normal circumstances.

In the thoracic spine, normal motion measured 60° of total flexion and extension, 60° of total lateral bending and 30° of total rotation. Despite the fact that all braces tested were lumbar braces, they all had some effect on thoracic motion. Saggital motion was most reduced by the molded TLSO with 49% restriction, followed by the Camp corset at

33%, while the Raney Jacket and elastic corset only provided 16% restriction. The Raney Jacket and the molded TLSO also provided the most restriction in lateral bending and rotation.

Table I consists of the free motion present in the lumbar and thoracic spines as well as the reduction with each brace tested.

LUMBAR

Brace	Fl. & Ext.	Tot. Lat.	Tot. Rot.
None	70 + 39	31 + 21	8 + 12
Raney	15 + 17	6 + 16 (81%)	-
Molded TLSO	22 + 15 (69%)	2 + 3 (97%)	-
Camp Corset	33 + 17 (53%)	8 + 9 (79%)	-
Elastic	48 + 31 (31%)	12 + 10 (61%)	-

THORACAL

Brace	Fl. & Ext.	Lat. Tot.	Rot. Tot.
None	49 + 69	60 + 31	90 + 30
Raney	41 + 32	38 + 35	35 + 35 (61%)
Molded TLSO	25 + 20 (49%)	37 + 19 (38%)	36 + 14 (60%)
Camp Corset	41 + 20 (16%)	53 + 12 (12%)	64 + 25 (39%)
Elastic	33 + 32 (33%)	52 + 30 (12%)	55 + 21 (29%)

This data reveals that all braces significantly ($p<.05$) restricted free lumbar and thoracic motion in the sagittal (flexion and extension) and frontal (left and right lateral bending) planes. The normal unrestricted motion encompassed a large range of variation. This wide range also exists with the data associated with the braces tested.

All subjects rated the comfort of each brace after testing. The elastic corset was rated 9.3; the Camp corset 7.3; the molded TLSO 4.2, and the Raney Jacket 2.1. When comparing the elastic corset and the Raney Jacket the p value was $<.05$. This verifies that there is an inverse relationship between a brace's ability to restrict motion and comfort.

Discussion

This study analyzed the degree of restriction provided by four lumbar braces. All braces were additionally evaluated for comfort. The Raney Jacket provided maximal restriction but was also the most uncomfortable brace tested, and therefore, the least acceptable. The most comfortable and accepted brace was the elastic corset which was the least restrictive of all braces tested. These findings must be considered when balancing patient compliance with the amount of immobilization that is necessary for a particular condition. The prescriber must determine how much and what type of immobilization is required as well as the degree of comfort that is provided by each brace, since patient compliance is an important factor in prescribing an orthosis.

References

Chapman, C., Casey, K., Dubner, R., Foley, K. & Gracely, R. 1985; Reading, A. Pain 22, 1.

Dorsky, S., Buchalter, D., Kahanowitz, N. & Nordin, M., 1986, A Noninvasive Technique forExamining Spinal Motion. Presented at the International Society for Study of the Lumbar Spine, (Abstract).

Hanley, E., Matteri, R. & Frymoyer, J. 1976, Accurate Roentgenographic Determination of LumbarFlexion-Extension. Clinical Orthopaedic and Related Research. 115, 145.

Macrae, J. & Wright, V., 1969, Measurement of Back Movement. Annual of Rheumatic Diseases, 28, 584.

Moll. J. & Wright, V., 1969, Normal Range of SpinalMobility.Annualof Rheumatic Diseases. 28, 584.

Morris, J., 1974, Low Back Brace. Clinical Orthopaedic Related Research. 102, 126.

Norton, P. & Brown, T., 1957, The Immobilizing Efficiency of Back Braces. Journal of Bone and Joint Surgery, 39A, 111.

Perry, J., 1970, The Use of External Support in the Treatment of Low Back Pain. Journal of Bone and Joint Surgery, 52A, 1440.

Portck, I., 1983, Correlation Between Radiographic and Clinical Measurement of Lumbar Spine Movement. British Journal of Rheumatology, 22, 197.

Three Space Tracher, Users Manual, McDonnell Douglas ElectronicCompany, Colchester, Vermont 05446 1985.

THE USE OF THE HETTINGER TEST
IN PRE-EMPLOYMENT SCREENING

D. Thompson, A. Lowerson, M. Zalewski

DEPARTMENT OF ENGINEERING PRODUCTION
UNIVERSITY OF BIRMINGHAM

Abstract

As part of an on-going research programme into the recognition of causes and prevention of occupationally related musculo-skeletal disorders, the Hettinger test is being examined on a test-retest-retest basis. Preliminary findings suggest it is insufficiently reliable and valid for use as a pre-employment screening test for tenosynovitis.

Introduction

Pre-employment Screening

In industries where a high incidence of Tenosynovitis exists amongst the workforce, any test which could show a predisposition to injury and be administered as a pre-employment screening test would clearly be of great value both in terms of the avoidance of personal injury and the subsequent socio-economic cost. Conversely, if a properly administered test is neither reliable nor valid a section of the population could be precluded from employment which in times of high unemployment could bring about equal socio-economic suffering.

Tests for Predisposition

Hettinger (1957) extended his earlier work (Hettinger & Beck, 1956) on the susceptibility of miners to mechanical stress to develop a test for predisposition for stenographers and punch card operators. The test was based on physiological observations that mechanical vibration of the hand causes vasoconstriction followed by vasodilation when vibration ceases, and that this can be measured by the fall in skin temperature and subsequent rise on the back of the hand.

The Hettinger index takes into account hand temperature before and after vibration and the time required before return to the initial base line. An index was calculated from the formula:-

$$\text{Index}(I) = \frac{1 + t}{1 + T} \left(1 + \frac{Z}{4}\right)$$

Where t = maximum drop in skin temperature

T = maximum rise in skin temperature in 5 minutes

z = time taken in minutes to regain original skin temperature (temps °C)

The index may have values increasing from zero but Hettinger (1958) noted index values below 1.3 seldom indicates predisposition, values between 1.3 and 1.6 are uncertain in their prediction and that only values over 1.6 predict with any great probability a predisposition to Tenosynovitis.

From his studies he suggested that its use was 80% successful in differentiating between the susceptible and non-susceptible. The work was later repeated by other scientists. The findings of Welch (1973) and Sakurai (1977) are consistent in agreement, and to a lesser extent is Schroter (1967). However, completely contrary results were obtained by Kuorinka et al (1981).

The Hettinger test in screening

Kuorinka concluded that the index value appeared to be dependent on the temperature of the test room, together with the possible interaction of the thermal balance, and was of "no value in screening for predisposition to tenosynovitis in an occupational health setting". And that, because intra-individual variation is so great no inferences can be made on the basis of one screening test. This study examines the reliability of the test on a test-retest basis when carried out in a controlled environment.

Method

Apparatus

The Hettinger vibrator consists of a wooden ball 65mm in diameter which vibrates at a frequency of 50Hz with an amplitude of 2mm. During vibration the ball is depressed by subjects with a force of 5 kg.

Room temperature was monitored constantly during the tests and was controlled at $18.5\,°C \pm 0.5\,°C$.

Hand skin temperature was measured using a Comark electronic thermometer with the sensor taped between the first and second meta-carpels on the dorsum of the preferred hand.

Subjects

Seven males and eight females - age range 22-38.

Test Procedure

As a pretest instruction, subjects were required to abstain from vigorous exercise, taking hot drinks and smoking for two hours before the test. The tests took place atweekly intervals on the same day and time over a three week period.

The subjects were seated throughout the tests and following the fixing of the temperature sensor to the hand, the hand was rested on a wooden block and monitoring took place until skin temperature had stabilized to within $\pm$ 0.1 °C over consecutive minutes. When this stability had been reached, subjects depressed the ball on the apparatus with a force of 5 kg and the hand was vibrated for 30 seconds, the hand was then returned to its resting position.

Skin temperature was recorded every 5 seconds for the first 30 seconds following vibration, then every 10 seconds for 5 minutes, then at 30 second intervals until the base-line level had been regained, or until 15 minutes had elapsed.

Results

Table I. The tenosynovitis index values of fifteen subjects performing three repeated trials.

Subject	Trials		
	1	2	3
1	4.8	2.12	2.42
2	2.75	0.65	1.07
3	1.15	1.02	1.17
4	1.98	0.88	0.99
5	1.15	0.82	1.15
6	2.58	1.07	2.92
7	3.65	1.46	0.83
8	0.95	1.47	3.72
9	1.58	1.15	1.89
10	2.94	2.59	0.99
11	3.24	5.91	4.55
12	2.5	1.75	2.17
13	0.83	0.97	1.6
14	2.37	1.2	1.0
15	1.04	0.81	0.96

Table 2. Tenosynovitis Index Test Consistency.

Subject	Trial 1 P	Trial 1 N.P.	Trial 2 P	Trial 2 N.P.	Trial 3 P	Trial 3 N.P.
1	x		x		x	
2	x			x		x
3		x		x		x
4	x			x		x
5		x		x		x
6	x			x	x	
7	x			x		x
8		x		x	x	
9		x		x	x	
10	x		x			x
11	x		x		x	
12	x		x		x	
13		x		x	x	
14	x			x		x
15		x		x		x

P = Index >1.6 = predisposition
NP = Index <1.6 = no predisposition

Conclusions

In controlled conditions three of our subjects scored consistently above the index value and three consistently below. However, the remaining nine had values both above and below the index values on successive trials.

Doubt already exists concerning the validity of the test to predict a predisposition to tenosynovitis and a longitudinal study will be required to provide further proof. However, in addition to this one must consider the reliability of the test as shown by the inconsistency of the test-retest index values. Because of this, the test can not be recommended as a pre-employment screening test for tenosynovitis.

References

Hettinger T.H., Beck W. 1956, Der Einfluss sinusforminger sehwingungen auf die Skelemuskolatur. International Zeitschrift fur Physiologie und Arbeitsphysiologie 16: 250-264.

Hettinger T.H. 1957 Ein Test zur Erkennung der Disposition zu Schnenscheidenentzundungen. International Zeitschrift fur angewandt Physiologie ensclessende Arbeitsphysiologie 16: 472-479.

Kuorinka I, Videman T, Lepisto M 1981 Reliability of a vibration test in screening for predisposition to tenosynovitis. European Journal of Applied Physiology 47: 356-376.

Sakurai T 1977 Vibration effects on hand arm system. Pt.2 Observations of skin temperature. Industrial Health 15: 59-66.

Schroter G 1967 Zur eignung des hettinger-testes fur die erkennung der disposition zu uberlast ungsschaden. Intermittent Archiv fur Gewerbepathologie und Gewerbehygine 23: 99-105.

Welch R 1973 The measurement of physiological predisposition to tenosynovitis. Ergonomics 16: 665-668.

REDUCING UPPER LIMB STRAIN INJURY BY REDESIGN:
A CASE STUDY IN THE FOOD PROCESSING INDUSTRY

M.H. Mabey, A.J. Pethick, R.J. Graves and P.K. Adams*

Ergonomics Branch, Institute of Occupational Medicine,
c/o British Coal HQ Technical Department,
Stanhope Bretby, Burton-on-Trent, Staffs DE15 OQD

*UB Frozen Foods Limited, Thame, Oxon.

SUMMARY

Two strategies may be adopted to reduce upper limb strain injury, the organisational and redesign strategies. The former includes selection, training, trainee probation, job rotation, or provision of physiotherapy, and in the extreme case withdrawal from the industrial activity in which the problem arises. The latter includes changes in specific work practices, rearrangement of workplaces, improvements to tools and other equipment, or selective automation of process elements. Accounting procedures currently in use do not tend to highlight costs incurred in adopting the organisational strategy, whereas those incurred in redesign are clearly ascribable.

This paper describes an ergonomic approach to cost-effective redesign which sought to limit the effects of upper limb strain injuries by eradicating their suspected causes.

INTRODUCTION

In the two years prior to the study, there had been an increase in wrist and arm problems apparently associated with the chicken processing tasks. When the number of employees apparently exhibiting symptoms of tenosynovitis became relatively large, exclusion on medical grounds from performing manipulative tasks made manning those tasks very difficult, resulting in loss of production. To overcome this, and to reduce the incidence of health problems, the management adopted an organisational strategy. A code of practice was established dealing with procedures for recruitment, health education for recruits, training, and the treatment and rehabilitation of tenosynovitis sufferers.

The process under consideration was the butchering of chicken carcasses which had been slaughtered, drawn and chilled off-site, and preparation of oven-ready chicken portions for a retail chain. The main tasks in this process were dismembering, skinning, boning-off, slicing, stuffing, freezing, frying and packing. Many of the tasks involved manipulation or use of knives. The workforce of 400-450 was predominantly female, and about 75% were employed in the butchery room.

A rotation system was devised for workers in the butchery room, allowing flexibility of manning to accommodate rehabilitation, training and cover for absence due to sickness or holidays. A two-hourly change resulted in each worker having four different tasks during the working day, alternating between tasks assessed by the management as being of high or low risk in terms of upper limb strain, based on the frequency and intensity of hand and arm movements required. Because many of the tasks were in the high risk category, each employee spent at least half the time on high risk tasks.

When all these measures had been put into operation, occurrences of tenosynovitis stabilised, but did not diminish as had been hoped. The factory management realised that redesign of butchery tasks would be necessary in order to achieve any reduction.

APPROACH USED IN THE REDESIGN PROCESS

The management intended to integrate several tasks to increase task diversity and reduce the overall risk level of the integrated task with respect to upper limb strain. The Institute of Occupational Medicine was asked to evaluate the loads imposed by individual tasks and by the integrated task. Experienced operators were observed performing tasks at normal production speed. The method used, reported elsewhere in these proceedings (Pethick et al, 1987), consisted of objective measures of posture, particularly for the elbow and wrist joints, of activity rate and duration, of the workspace, and of operator anthropometry. The tools observed in use were also assessed with respect to their possible contribution to upper limb strain injuries. Whole body and regional discomfort questionnaires were administered.

The tasks being considered for integration were boning-off breasts, weighing and trimming, slicing, and stuffing. The management had suspected that boning-off was a high risk task. This was confirmed as a result of the ergonomic investigation, which also demonstrated that it was unsuitable for integration with any of the other three tasks under consideration, due in particular to the type of posture required and the rate of knife wear. Use of the knife in this task blunted the edge quickly but it did not need to be kept very sharp, whereas in slicing the knife had to be as sharp as possible but was not rapidly blunted. If these two tasks were integrated the knives would have to be sharpened much more frequently, adding to the workload and increasing expenditure on knives. Having more than one knife at each workstation was impractical for safety and hygiene reasons.

Weighing and trimming appeared to be a low risk task given the carcass weights at the time of observation, but it was noted that the frequency of movements and the task cycle time would be markedly affected by any increase in carcass weight, a factor dependent on availability from suppliers. Here again, the pattern of knife wear was incompatible with the sharpness required in slicing.

Whereas slicing was considered to be at the lower end of the range of high risk tasks, stuffing was at the upper end of the low risk range and had many ergonomic features in common with slicing but no conflicting requirements. These two tasks could therefore be combined, with the benefit of reducing the static load imposed by gripping the knife over a two hour period in the separate slicing task.

Task synthesis based on the ergonomic data showed that integration of all four tasks would probably result in a high risk task. This was due to factors such as the whole-body postures required for boning-off which would be unsatisfactory for the other tasks and the knives would rapidly become too blunt for slicing. Also, the amount of equipment in the workspace would hamper reach to the conveyor used to deliver chickens and remove stuffed breasts. These and other issues rendered it an unsatisfactory arrangement. It was concluded that no integration should take place until improvements to the equipment and workspace had been undertaken. Tasks excluded from the initial survey would also have to be studied to assess the full effect of integration as this might restrict the range of jobs that other employees could undertake.

ANALYSIS OF SYSTEM REQUIREMENTS

The company had accepted that any successful redesign strategy would be likely to include automation of the most stressful elements of tasks and improvements to existing equipment if automation proved impracticable. The dismembering and skinning tasks which immediately preceded boning-off had already been identified as highly stressful tasks which could be partially automated. The Institute provided expertise on ergonomic issues within a specially formed working team responsible for implementing the automation, equipment redesign and other task design changes that were being proposed.

The working team set criteria for acceptability of any changes to the methods of production, based on manufacturing targets, manning levels, continued use of the established rotation system, and adherence to ergonomic principles. In order to identify problems prior to implementation, the Institute constructed a system diagram of the proposed arrangements. Individual tasks were examined as modules to ensure compatibility between input and output requirements of adjacent modules. Two potential bottlenecks in production were identified where the new tasks would be unlikely to achieve production and stress reduction objectives at the intended manning levels. These problems would be resolved by employing an additional part-time operator at one location and by improving the equipment configuration at the other.

The system analysis revealed that responsibility for knife sharpening was not formally allocated to particular personnel, and no specific procedure had been established to ensure that knives were kept as sharp as needed to optimise quality, productivity and minimise forces applied by the operators. The practice was for operators to request a supervisor to sharpen knives when they judged it necessary. The operator would continue working with a second knife while the first was being sharpened. Although this was effective and acceptable within the existing system of working, knife sharpening would have to be reviewed as an important formal component of any new working arrangement.

Analysis clearly showed that boning-off could require thorough redesign to achieve the desired stress reduction. Adding another task to boning-off would have advantages in reducing upper limb strain injury risk provided that the operator put down the knife as much as possible. Incorporating an activity with commercial benefit was preferable, such as one involving recovery or use of wishbone meat. With this possibility in mind, a cone support for boning-off was evaluated. This device improved the angle of presentation of the bird to the operator. The forces involved in wishbone removal were assessed, as well as the posture required, any constraints on technique and especially the muscle loads and posture imposed by the special tool used for wishbone removal.

Wrist movement could be minimised by improving knife

design. The most satisfactory angle of the knife handle in relation to the blade in the cone boning-off task was determined by simulation. Provision of an angled tool holder would encourage operators to pick up the wishbone tool or boning knife as late as possible in the cycle and to put them down as early as possible. The supervisor would need to ensure that working heights were correctly adjusted in the early stages, until boners-off made the correct adjustments habitually. The frequency of occurrence of wrist movement and the range of wrist deviation in both hands were substantially reduced in the simulated task. With other improvements in general posture and workspace layout, boning-off would become a relatively low risk task.

Changing boning-off workspaces would prevent operators from reaching across the conveyor belt, so the skinning machine operator would have to place the birds on the belt on the correct side for each boning-off operator. This could be achieved by improving the skinning equipment configuration, which was also simulated to derive detailed design requirements.

From the analysis of the system diagram and simulations, it was concluded that the redesign of the skinning and boning-off tasks would not affect subsequent operations. However, porterage would be affected in two ways:

(i) the deeper boning-off work surface would reduce the width of the access corridor;
(ii) increasing the number of carcass disposal bins, ensuring that each boner-off had easy access to a bin, would impose an additional task demand on the porters.

ASSESSING STRAIN INJURY REDUCTION

Although the proposed task and equipment changes are not yet fully implemented, monitoring of the effects of changes has begun. The intention is to compare the rate and distribution of upper limb strain incidence and recurrence with the situation before organisational changes were made, and with the situation after apparent containment of the problem by organisational means. The results from this comparison will be reported in due course.

It may not be possible to distinguish effects brought about by different redesign changes, since the sample population is rather small for statistical comparison and the changes have been introduced during changes in the products of the factory. However, it would be useful for the management to have some estimate of the relative contribution of each change as a basis for assignment of priorities for action, within this company or others in its group, especially if funds were limited.

CONCLUSIONS

Equipment and task redesign are expected to be effective in reducing upper limb strain problems because probable causes were addressed such as posture, forces, static loads and ranges of movement, rather than attempting to ameliorate the effects. The ultimate success of these changes will be assessed over time, but interim impressions indicate that this approach has been both successful and cost-effective in easing the introduction of new equipment and processes to the factory.

In order to respond rapidly and effectively to the problem of upper limb strain injury the company required the study to be carried out and reported as quickly as possible. The findings had to be readily understood by the management so that decisions could be based on them. Budgetary constraints emphasised the need for inexpensive techniques to be applied and for consultancy expenses to be kept to the minimum consistent with acceptable depth of investigation. The study was carried out with the management's objectives and constraints in mind so that the information provided was appropriate to their requirements. This was achieved by maximising the use of local skills. For example, where possible, simulation studies and on-site measurement were carried out by the Company personnel with guidance from the ergonomists. Tool prototype manufacture was carried out in a similar way.

From the approach adopted, the management developed an awareness of ergonomic factors which kept discussion of detail to a minimum. This also ensured that ergonomic principles would continue to be applied after completion of the immediate project without direct involvement of ergonomists.

REFERENCE

Pethick, A.J., Mabey, M.H. & Graves, R.J., 1987, Development of a Practical Method for Workplace Redesign to Reduce Upper Limb Strain Injury. In: Proceedings of Musculoskeletal Disorders at Work. Surrey: Robens Institute.

REDUCING REPITITIVE STRAIN AND BACK PAIN
AMONG BRICKLAYERS

Noah K. Akinmayowa

Ergonomics Division, Department of Psychology,
University of Lagos

ABSTRACT

In this paper, Medical data and case studies on the prevalence of musculo-skeletal disorders among bricklayers are discussed. From ergonomic study of the work, it was observed that repitive strain and back-pain that were found to be highly prevalent in the industry can be reduced through the application of ergonomic principles to improve work methods, and work structuring.

INTRODUCTION

In Nigeria, Medical data on the prevalence of musculo-skeletal disorders among occupational groups are limited, due to lack of co-ordinated research. Extensive study of the problems of occupational hazards in order to improve occupational health schemes through the introduction of ergonomic improvements is desirable.

This study was undertaken to identify the health problems of bricklayers who carry out their jobs in hot/humid climatic conditions and employ inadequate posture for a very long working period.

METHODS

Medical Survey: Medical records on the prevalence of musculo-skeletal disorders among bricklayers were surveyed from case histories of 6,500 men; self employed (N = 4,300) and those employed by large construction firms (N = 2,200).

The data represented returns from 38 Medical practitioners who were randomly selected and approached for informations that were only useful to epidemiological surveys.

The selection criteria ensured the representation of rural and urban bricklayers who perform the construction of houses, bridges and drainage systems

Job Factors and Subjective Assessment of Comfort/Discomfort:

From the sample (N = 6,500) random selection of 1,500 subjects was made. They were requested to respond to a questionnaire designed to evaluate job factors affecting worker health. Subjective assessment of comfort/discomfort of body parts arising from the job performance was obtained from the subjects using the method adopted by Corlett and Bishop 1976.

Task Analysis:

For task analysis, three groups were selected consisting of 60 bricklayers who suffer significantly higher prevalence of musculo-skeletal disorders of backpain and repititive strain.

They consisted of those who build houses (N=24) bridges (N=20) and drainage systems (N=16). The average number of years on the job was 10.5 $\pm$ 3.1 years.

The distribution of the study period enable each individual/group to be studied once a week for a total period of 7 weeks. The bricklaying tasks were recorded on video for four hours representing random selection of major tasks which were carried out during a full eight hour working period.

Preceived Factors and Efforts:

At the end of each recording, subjects selected from a list, factors which negatively or positively influenced their performance. Part of the list was similar to those employed by Pateman and Clark (1986). Perceived efforts on specific tasks were obtained from each subject with the Perceived Exertion Scale of Borg (1970).

RESULTS

Musculo-skeletal disorders was found to be prevalent in the bricklaying industry affecting 97% of the bricklayers. In these subjects (N = 6,305), the severity of the disorder increased with age since in subjects below 27 years (30%), musculoskeletal disorders was confined to the shoulder, arms, wrist, fingers and pain at the legs.

Serious musculo-skeletal disorders of lower back pain, repititive pain of the lumbar region were reported in bricklayers who are over 27 years. For older men aged above 45 years (30%), the disorder involved regular pain occuring every day and requiring medication or leave from work. Generally the prevalence of repititive strain was more for those who work in the bridge building industry (80%).

Although, general backpain, lower back pain shoulder pain, neck, arm and wrist pain were common problems, it was observed that 80% of the whole subjects identified loss in touch sensitivity in the finger as a major problem.

Those in the house construction were found to suffer from neck pain than for other groups.

It was shown that the rural bricklayers (40%) had a significantly higher prevalence of musculo-skeletal disorders than for the urban dwellers; $p < 0.005$, and $p < 0.05$ respectively.

From the questionnaire survey, which had response rate of 94%, factors which were indicated to affect health at work were related to the job load and stresses imposed by environmental heat stress. Movement and postural analysis showed that operators were static for considerable period of the time. The cycle time showed that 75% of the time the workers were involved in finishing job.

Perceived exertion scale was found to be influenced by work surface as workers who perform on Scaffolds judged their efforts as greater than for those who are on the ground when they perform similar task.

This was taken to be a factor of the strain/stresses imposed by the limited work space since scaffolding limited free movement.

Result of post-recording questionnaire showed that fatigue and heat stress was considered by subjects as factors limiting performance efforts.

DISCUSSION

On the full evaluation of the data, the high prevalence of musculo-skeletal disorders was established. The implications for the health of the individual are tremendous. The rationale for a healthy workforce imply that the trend should be checked since there are economic implications. The need for occupational health specialist to direct energy at reducing musculo-skeletal disorders in this job become very important. The relevant factors influencing performance are the age, job type and environment. All these has ergonomic implications.

Rural dwellers do not have opportunities for adequate medical care and this was attributed to the high prevalance of musculo-skeletal disorders than in urban areas.

It was felt that the introduction of ergonomic principles in planning rest period, work structuring and schedules will enable workers perceive objective efforts in group performance to eliminate misconception about rewards on the job. Job evaluation in this industry is of importance for industrial peace in the union.

CONCLUSION

The study reveal the occupational hazards of bricklayers with reference to areas in the job, that exert considerable pressure in the performance of tasks.

It is expected that ergonomic efforts at improving the work situation will reduce the hazards.

Acknowledgements

I would like to thank the Department of Occupational Health of the Federal Ministry of Health, Lagos, for encouragements and administrative support.

REFERENCES

Borg, G. A. V., 1970, Perceived exertion as an indicator of somatic stress. Scandinavian Journal of Rehabilitation Medicine. 2 : 92 - 98.

Corlett, E. N. and Bishop, R. P., 1976, A technique For Assessing Postural Discomfort. Ergonomics, 19, 2, 175 - 182.

Pateman C. M. and Clark A. G., 1986, The Effects of Origin and Placement Sites on Repititive Handling Tasks. In Contemporary Ergonomics. Edited by D. J. Oborne (Proceedings of the Ergonomics Society's Annual Conference) Taylor & Francis Publications. 228.

MUSCULOSKELETAL DISORDERS AMONG CARGO HANDLERS

Noah K. Akinmayowa and Isaac Akintunji*

Ergonomics Division, Department of Psychology,
University of Lagos

*NAA Clinic, Nigeria Airport Authority, Ikeja

ABSTRACT

Ergonomic study of cargo handling was undertaken to investigate causes of Musculoskeletal disorders. It was observed that harzards contributing to the reported disorders arise from the strains and stresses of Manual Loading and unloading of Cargoes, the problems of equipment useage and reliability and the non-application of ergonomic principles to job performance where necessary.

In order to reduce occupational hazards, ergonomic improvements were recommended.

INTRODUCTION

The ergonomist was invited by the Medical Consultant to investigate causes of the increase in musculoskeletal disorders of back-pain and repititive strain among cargo handlers since musculoskeletal disorders were clinical reasons for the absence from work of 30% of the workforce every week for a period of six months. Detailed ergonomic study of cargo handling activities was carried out with the following objectives:

* to analyse the processes in the performance of job.
* to determine the effectiveness of the processes.

* to identify the problems which lead to musculoskeletal disorders.
* to eliminate the problems through the introduction of ergonomic techniques necessary for a safe satisfying and productive processes.

METHODS

The research team obtained the full cooperation of the Management and workforce since the health problems were established.

Method and time study techniques were used for the ergonomic analysis.

For this purpose, Cargo handling activities carried out by Thirty men who were divided into 6 groups (N=5 per group), were recorded on video. Each film took 150 minutes, covering the entire locations in the workplace.

Each group was randomly assigned to shifts for the study, per day for a total of 21 days.

Throughout the video recording, heart rate of all the subjects were simultaneously and continuously recorded using the Telemetry technique.

In order to establish the time taken for vital processes of the job which involve cargo search, lifting, loading, unloading and transportation, time study was carried out in addition to the construction of Flow process and Simultaneous Motion Cycle charts.

This study also include an examination of workplace layout of actual dimensions and sketches to enable the identification of necessary structural adjustments, which will be ideal for job performance.

A questionnaire which was designed to survey attitudes of workers to their job and workplace and assess suggestions at improving the work-job-environment interactions was administered to Cargo Handlers (N=30), Supervisors (N=3) and Personnel Managers (N=8).

RESULTS

The video recordings were analysed with a technique of Holzmann (1982) to identify the processes and efforts for the cargo handling task.

From the analysis five main problems areas were identified during the cargo handling operations.

1. Long Distance in the Workplace

    The workplace covered an area between the aircraft stand and warehouse. It was observed that operators mannually push and pull cages over long distances.

2. Poor Accessibility

    As a result of poor accessibility along the route to the warehouse operators are forced to manoeuver cages over rough floor surface and the risks to accidents of slip and fall were observed.

3. Cargo Identification

    Cargoes were not properly identifiable regarding the weight categories. Heavy cargoes were difficult to handle as loading/unloading activities were difficult and involve introduction of trial and error tactics by operators.

    Due to lack of information on cargo weight, cages were often overloaded and difficult to move.

4. Equipment Usage and Reliability

    It was observed that existing cages for transporting cargoes are not adequately maintained. Since the job is predominantly manual, a lot of effort was required to push or pull cages with stiff wheel over rough floor surfaces.

5. Ergonomic Problem

    The analysis show that operators do not apply

ergonomic principles to job processes such as
in lifting which represented 75% of the work
process. It was observed that operators perform
pushing activities than pulling activities
during the transportation process from aircraft
stand to warehouse.

As a result of the identification of these problems,
desirable ergonomic improvements for the workplace,
job performance, equipment and organization were
recommended

1. Workplace

   It was stressed that transportation within the
   workplace should be limited through the reduction
   of the distance since the job is predominantly
   manual. The need for adequate maintenance of
   workplace floor surface was stressed in order
   to eliminate the friction between it and the
   wheel of the cages. Hazards of slip and fall
   must be removed. The introduction of schemes
   such as music-while-you work should be carried
   out.

2. Job Performance

   Operators should endeavour to introduce variation
   in posture and ergonomic principles during the
   lifting processes. This can be achieved through
   training. In the transportation of cages,
   operators should alternate between pulling and
   pushing cages. Whenever possible, cages should
   be pulled most of the time, for physiological
   reasons since heart rates were lower in the latter.

3. Equipment

   The equipment (cages) must be adequately maintained to improve carriage capacity of large
   cargoes. This will minimise the stress and
   strains when operators manipulate and manoeuver
   large cargoes into cages that are inadequate
   for such sizes.

4. Organization

   Operators must be encouraged to report cases of illhealth in the course of work as early as possible and management must encourage worker participation in selecting work shifts and schedules.

DISCUSSION

The cost-benefit analysis of these improvement were accepted by management and considerable improvement of 65% reduction in disorders of the musculoskeletal regions were reported 2 months after implementation. This trend is expected to improve.

The result has shown the use of ergonomic analysis to improve human work activities. The simplicity of the procedure is an advantage with regard to its general application.

Since 86% of cargo handling task was spent lifting, pulling and pushing activities, it became obvious that considerable pressure will be exerted on the trunk flexion. Pressure on the trunk flexion was reported by Nicholson et al (1986), to be greater for pushing than pulling loaded cages.

It was also reported (Lagercrans 1984) that a 55% to 100% increase in the force required to push poorly maintained cages in comparison to new ones. It was believed that recommendation of adequate maintenance of cages in the present study will be useful.

The application of ergonomic principles to posture changes and a safe workplace layout has very positive implications and worker participation as an integral part of improving decision-making process in organization has long been highly recognised.

CONCLUSION

The benefits of ergonomic principles in cargo handling activities are illustrated for the benefits of worker and management in the provision of optimum man-work-environment system relationships.

Acknowledgements

We would like to thank all the workforce of the cargo handling department of the Nigeria Airport Authority and the Department of Electronics Engineering, University of Lagos for technical support.

REFERENCES

Holzmann. P., 1982, ARBAN - A new method for analysis of ergonomic effort. <u>Applied Ergonomics</u>, 13.2, 82-86.

Lagercrans, S., 1984, Quoted in Nicholson et al (1986) Handling problems associated with the distribution of supplies. In <u>contemporary Ergonomics</u>. Edited by D. J. Oborne (Proceedings of the Ergonomics Society's Annual Conference) Taylor & Francis Publications•235.

Nicholson, A. S., Ridd, J. E. and Fernandes, A. F., Handling Problems associated with the distribution of supplies. In <u>contemporary Ergonomics</u>. Edited by D. J. Oborne (Proceedings of the Ergonomics Society's Annual Conference) Taylor & Francis Publications 232 - 236.

AN INTERNATIONAL COMPARISON OF THE PREVALENCE OF RSI AMONG KEYBOARD OPERATORS AND ITS RELATIONSHIP TO OFFICE WORK PRACTICES

GABRIELE BAMMER

Director's Section, Research School of Social Sciences, Australian National University, GPO Box 4 Canberra, ACT 2601, Australia

While repetition strain injuries (RSI) are well recognised in most countries, there have been no international comparisons of the incidence or prevalence of these disorders. Negotiations to establish such an international study are underway, and the results of a pilot study examining the feasibility of international comparisons are reported here.

University office staff in departments of History and Physics in Australia, Japan, England, Germany, Sweden, Canada and the United States of America were interviewed.

They were asked about any experience they had had with RSI. Information was also sought about the characteristics of their work, including task diversity, work history, details about keyboard work, work organisation and job satisfaction. Most workers also filled out a time sheet of their activities for one day.

Interesting differences were found between countries, not only in the prevalence of RSI, but also in office work practices. The association between these two factors will be discussed.

ACKNOWLEDGEMENTS

I am indebted to the following people for arranging interviews for me: in Japan, H. Aoyama, T. Itani, T. Kondo, M. Miyao & R. Tokunaga; in England, W.N. Trethowan; in Germany, A. Cakir; in Sweden, G. Johansson; in Canada, J.T. Purdham; and in the USA, M.J. Smith, K. Miezio & T.J. Armstrong.

I am especially grateful to Dr Masaru Miyao for translating my questionnaire into Japanese and to the abovementioned Japanese colleagues who acted as interpreters.

INTEGRATED BIOMECHANICAL EXAMINATION OF THE
MUSCULOSKELETAL SYSTEM

Dr. David Byfield

Anglo-European College of Chiropractic,
Parkwood Road,
Bournemouth,
BH5 2DF

   The medical, social, and economic impact of musculoskeletal dysfunction (MSD) has been well documented in
recent years (Cassidy et al 1985, Burton 1986). The impact
of musculoskeletal pain especially low back pain (LBP) has
been described as enormous and very costly (Nachemson 1976,
Kelsey 1979, Andersson 1981, Andersson 1981, Troup 1981,
Kelsey 1982, Lee et al 1985). Back pain appears to be the
most common presenting complaint within the musculoskeletal system (MSS) (Greenman 1985, Kirkaldy-Willis 1985),
and appears to have universal occurance as one of the major
causes of long term disability and loss of earnings in all
civilized societies (Diakow & Cassidy 1984). In fact,
Cassidy et al (1985) states that there is little doubt that
LBP affects the quality of life for just about everyone in
contemporary Western society. The magnitude of this problem
is clearly indicated when almost 80% of the general
population will experience LBP during their lifetime
(Brunarski 1982, White 1982, White & Gordon 1982, Kirkaldy-
Willis 1985).
   The etiology of spinal pain remains obscure and in most
cases unknown (Nachemson 1976, White 1982, Diakow & Cassidy
1984, Cassidy et al 1985, Kirkaldy-Willis 1985). It has
been reported that between 20 and 85% of LBP is diagnosed
as idiopathic (White 1982). To date the best medical
evaluation has been unable to determine the cause of LBP
precisely (White 1982).
   Why, then, does such a large proportion of LBP have no
definite etiology? One of the major problems with MSD lies
within the diagnosis (Kirkaldy-Willis 1979, Brunarski 1982,
Greenman 1985, Kirkaldy-Willis 1985), creating a situation
where effective intervention remains highly problematic
(Greenman 1985, Kirkaldy-Willis 1985). Therefore, since

an accurate diagnosis is a prerequisite, we should focus more attention on identifying the mechanical fault and less on the disease process itself (Greenman 1985). Kirkaldy-Willis (1979) states that treatment is usually given before the diagnosis is ever made and that everyone receives the same treatment regardless of the specific mechanical lesions. It therefore becomes essential for the diagnosis to correlate the mechanical spinal problem, to the presenting complaint, and clinical picture (Méal 1977).

The problem, therefore, seems to lie within the ability to establish an accurate diagnosis (Kirkaldy-Willis 1979, Greenman 1985). This ability is complicated by the following specific points for consideration:

1. the complexity and variability of the MSS anatomically, biomechanically, and neurologically (Greenman 1985).

2. the concept of the three joint complex within the motor unit (Farfan 1973).

3. the difficulty in identifying the anatomical source of pain as overlap of innervation and pain patterns exhibit complexity as all tissues of the spine are capable of generating pain (O'Brien 1984, Hackett, 1957, Mooney & Robertson 1975, Feinstein 1977).

4. several distinct lesions commonly yield much the same symptoms complex (Kirkaldy-Willis 1979, 1985).

5. the spine is not appreciated as a whole organ of posture and movement, a complex biomechanical interrelationship (Valkenburg & Haanen 1982).

6. the nature of LBP is that it is common, self-limiting, and highly recurrent (Kirkaldy-Willis & Cassidy 1985).

7. very little is known at the present about how the back and spine move during normal movements (Pearcy as reported by Burton Meeting Reports 1986).

8. lack of objective measures of function to validate both diagnostic techniques and methods of treatment (Kirkaldy-Willis 1985) (Pearcy 1986).

Therefore, disorders of the MSS are a multi-factorial problem requiring a simple, comprehensive, organized approach to searching for mechanical faults in order to assist more directly in the determination of the cause of the dysfunction.

A more integrated biomechanical approach to the examination will enhance the concept of the dual diagnosis (Gitelman 1980, Grice 1980, Kirkaldy-Willis 1985), which defines: (1) more accurately the site of the actual lesion and (2) the stage reached in the degenerative process - dysfunction, instability, restabilisation (Kirkaldy-Willis 1983) based upon a biomechanical evaluation of the patient as a whole (Gitelman 1976). The dual diagnosis plus the formation of a clinical impression of the total health status yields enough information about the patient to begin a more directed therapeutic intervention to correct the biomechanical fault(s), manage the ongoing condition, and determine a more realistic prognosis.

The problem is no longer one of statics but one of a dynamically functional organism which should be examined with the same biomechanical respect. Therefore, it is of paramount importance to have a keen working knowledge of anatomy, physiology, biomechanics, and kinesiology of the spinal column and extremities before determination of normal and abnormal function can be made (West 1980). Knowledge of the quality and the quantity of movement of a particular area of the spine and how that interrelates during normal activities is essential in our understanding of MSD.

The examination that yields the greatest amount of information regarding the function or lack of function of the MSS, eliminating subjectivity and enhancing objectivity is a primary directive as each procedure should complement and cross check the others.

The integrated examination that is suggested is based upon a biomechanical model (Fligg 1985), incorporating the following specific areas:
1. Dynamic Plumbline analysis and posture evaluation (Fig. 1A and 1B).
2. Ranges of motion determination.
3. Gait analysis.
4. Physical examination.
5. Neurological examination.
6. Orthopaedic examination.
7. Dynamic motion palpation.
8. Static palpatory procedures.
9. Joint play/end feel/spring analysis.
10. Muscle testing (strength/length).
11. Functional radiograph determination.
12. Laboratory investigation.

Each distinct element of the examination is organised into several positions of approach including:
a) Standing
b) Sitting
c) Supine
d) Side
e) Prone

This particular approach ensures the evaluation of the MSS analysing interrelationships between bodily systems

Figure 1. Plumbline Postural Evaluation.

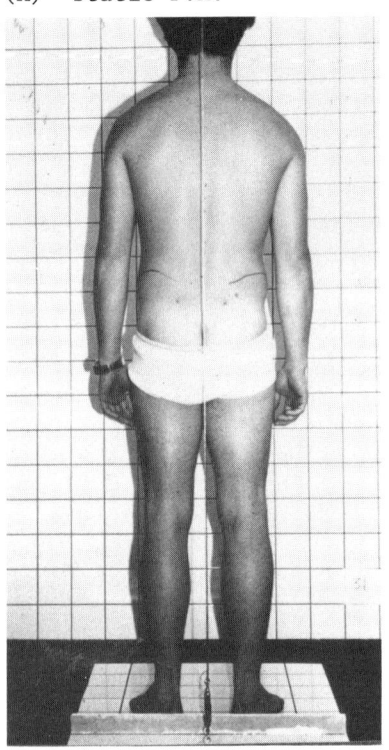

(A) Static P.A. (B) Dynamic Posture

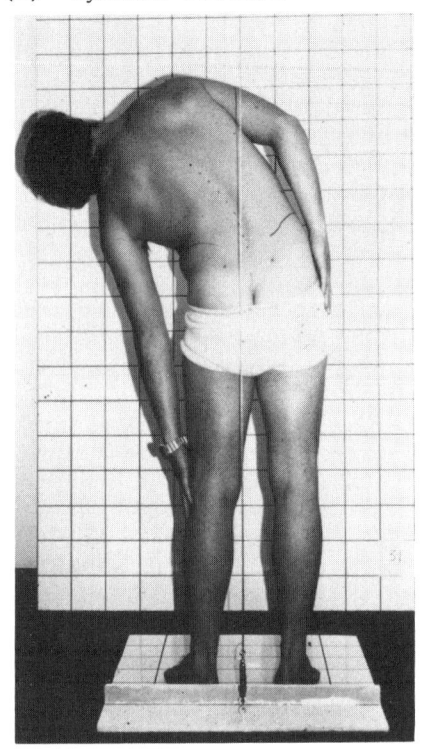

Figure 2. Clinical Integrated Examination Form: Examination Guide.

PHYSICAL EXAMINATION	INITIAL BP RT. LT.	SUBSEQUENT BP RT. LT.	PULSE PRESSURE RT. LT.	PULSE RATE RT. LT.
HEIGHT WEIGHT TEMP	RESP RATE LMP		G P	
Normals ✓ abnormals O	NO. OF CHILDREN		CR Cerebrum CB Cerebellum Roman Numeral Cranial Nerve Arabic Numeral Periph Nerve	

STANDING

GENERAL EXAMINATION
1. General Observation, Posture/Plumbline, Curvatures, Gait, Head, Shoulders, Pelvis, Hip, Knees, Ankle, Feet.
2. Height Weight

CHIROPRACTIC AND ORTHOPAEDIC EXAMINATION
3. Cervical; Active ROM, Flexion, Extension, Rotation, Lateral Flexion.
4. Shoulder; Active ROM, Apley's Scratch Tests
5. Lumbar; Active ROM, Flexion, Extension, Rotation, Lateral Flexion, Squat
6. Sacroiliac Motion Palpation Tests (5)

ORTHOPAEDIC TESTS
7. Adams, supported Adams
8. Kemps, compression, direct
9. Trendelenberg, straight leg raise test

NEUROLOGICAL
10. Heel Walking (L5), Toe Walking (SI)
11. Cerebellar; Rhomberg's, tandem gait, hopping, Underberger's etc.

SITTING

GENERAL EXAMINATION
12. Wetrim (CR)
13. Facial Expression (VII)
14. Voice (X), Phonation
15. Blood Pressures, pulses
16. Funduscopic examination
17. Respiration Rate; inspiration, expiration, expansion
18. Temperature
19. Thyroid, trachea, pulses, lympn nodes
20. Chest, heart, lungs, breast, axilla
21. Sinus (transilluminate), throat, nose, ear

CHIROPRACTIC AND ORTHOPAEDIC EXAMINATION
22. Jaw, Static and Motion Palpation end feel TMJ
23. Cervical; Passive, Active, Resisted ROM
24. Cervical; Static and Motion Palpation, end feel, Reclination Test (VBI)
25. Thoracic; Passive, Active, Resisted ROM
26. Thoracic; Static and Motion Palpation, end feel, RIB motion palpation, end feel
27. Lumbar; Passive, Active, Resisted ROM
28. Lumbar; Static and Motion Palpation, end feel
29. Shoulder, elbow, wrist, hands; inspection, palpation, ROM joint play, special tests (muscle girth, orthopaedic tests, pulses etc.)

ORTHOPAEDIC TESTS
30. Cervical Nerve Root; cervical compression, maximum cervical compression, shoulder depression, doorbell, distraction, shoulder abduction etc.
31. Thoracic Outlet; Adson's, Hyperabduction, Costoclavicular, Eden's
32. Lumbar; Kemp's, vertical compression, flip tests, Valsalva

NEUROLOGICAL
33. Cranial Nerves I-XII
34. Cerebellar; finger to nose, finger to finger, tap rhythm etc. Hautant's (VBI)
35. Deep Tendon and Superficial Reflexes
36. Sensation; Neck, Thorax, Upper Extremity, Lower Extremity; pain, temperature, discrimination, stereognosis etc
37. Muscle Strength (Various); dynamometer, objective, subjective (%) C5 Deltoid, C56 Biceps, C6 Wrist Extensors, C7 Wrist Flexors, Finger Extensors, C8 Finger Flexors, T1 Interossei

SUPINE

GENERAL EXAMINATION
38. Head and Neck; inspection, palpation, sinuses etc.
39. Chest; inspection, palpation etc.
40. Abdomen; inspection, auscultation, palpation, percussion

CHIROPRACTIC AND ORTHOPAEDIC EXAMINATION
41. Cervical; passive, resisted ROM
42. Cervical; static and motion palpation, end feel
43. Rib; palpate, spring, trigger points
44. Hip; ROM at 90° + 0°
45. Lower extremity; knee, ankle, foot, inspection, palpation, Rom, joint play, special tests (muscle girth, orthopaedic tests, pulses etc.)

ORTHOPAEDIC TESTS
46. SLR; Braggards, Bonnet's (SLR + int. rot.), SLR + ext. rot., Bowstring, WLR, Goldthwaites, modified Goldthwaites (SLR – neck flexion, Valsalva).
47. Gaenslen's; SI separation, SI compression
48. Thomas; Fabere Patrick (fig. 4) length and strength, Laguerre's (mod. fig. 4) Gauvains, Heel to Shin.

NEUROLOGICAL
49. Deep Tendon and Superficial Reflexes
50. VBI Tests; De Kleyn's.
51. Sensation; Neck, Thorax and Lower Extremity; pain, light touch temperature discrimination, vibration
52. Muscle Strength (Various); Objective, subjective (include sit-up). (%) L4 Quads, L5 Extensor Digitorum, S1 Peroneus Longus, S1 Plantar Flexion

SIDE

GENERAL EXAMINATION
53. Rectum and prostate

CHIROPRACTIC AND ORTHOPAEDIC EXAMINATION
54. Muscle Length; TFL, gluteus medius and minimus

ORTHOPAEDIC TESTS
55. Hip Abduction Stress, SI Compression

NEUROLOGICAL
56. Muscle Strength (Various); objective, subjective (%) (grade) QL (side leg, body), glut med, min, TFL

PRONE

GENERAL EXAMINATION
57. Kidney Punch

CHIROPRACTIC AND ORTHOPAEDIC TEST
58. Spinal + Rib Palpation; static palpation, joint play, spring, tenderness, hypertonicity, PA + LAT pressure test etc.
59. Pelvic Palpation; static and motion palpation, joint play; PSIS, iliolumbar lig., sacroiliac lig. sciatic notch, triggers
60. Spinal and Pelvic Percussion
61. Lower extremity (knee); Apley's grind and distract, and leg length

ORTHOPAEDIC TESTS
62. Knee Flexion; Ely's Sign (heel to buttock), Nachlas (femoral nerve stretch), Ely Heel to Buttock, Yeoman's, Hibb's, Homer Pheasant's (knee flexion provocation)

NEUROLOGICAL
63. Deep Tendon and superficial reflexes
64. Sensation, Thoracic, Pelvis, Upper and Lower Extremities pain, light touch, temperature, vibration
65. Muscle Strength; objective, subjective including chest raise). (%). (grade) quads, hams, glut max, hip rot

in all postural positions including weight bearing and non-weight bearing postures. The incorporation of a thorough case history and systems review is included to assist in understanding the etiological factors with respect to the functional disturbance.

We have developed at the Anglo-European College of Chiropractic a clinical teaching form (Fig. 2 & Fig. 3) to guide the examination and to function as a recording base which brings together all information pertinent to the case for the development of a diagnosis and clinical impression.

The essence of the examination is function and movement as the exam proceeds from an evaluation of posture to the analysis of the quality and quantity of periperal, pelvis, sacroiliac, and intervertebral joint movement based on a system of dynamic motion palpation (Fig. 4)(Gillet 1960, Mennel 1964, Maigne 1972, Cassidy & Potter 1978, Gitelman 1980, Grice 1980, Gillet & Liekens 1981, Fligg 1984). Static joint challenge as well as dynamic motion palpation methods determine normal and abnormal motion segment dynamics (Grice 1980). It has been suggested that it can be confirmed by dynamic radiographic examination (Cassidy 1976, Grice 1979, Kirkaldy-Willis 1985).

Motion palpation is based on the fact that a normal diarthroidial joint has a physiological range of motion (Fig. 5) in each plane of movement (flexion, extension, lateral bending, rotation and coupled motions)(Sandoz 1976). Analysis of each joint through its active passive joint play and end feel characteristics stresses the stabilising holding elements defined at that particular level of motion (Fig. 6).

The physical examination of the MSS must be conducted in the context of a complete physical examination of the whole patient. The objective is to determine functional capacity, in order to precipitate major mechanical faults and secondary compensatory mechanisms. Interpretation of standard orthopaedic tests should yield information not only about pain, but also valuable information regarding functional biomechanics. (Breig & Troup 1979). The work by Terret (1982), Pearcy (1986) amd Troup (1986) is necessary in order to biomechanically interpret these standard orthopaedic tests and measuring systems in order to enhance objectivity.

This paper presents the background and the elements of an integrated examination that should be at least considered to yield maximum information relative to the function of the spine, pelvis, and extremities in order that a more accurate diagnosis and clinical impression of the

Integrated biomechanical examination 207

Figure 3. Clinical Integrated Examination: Recording Base

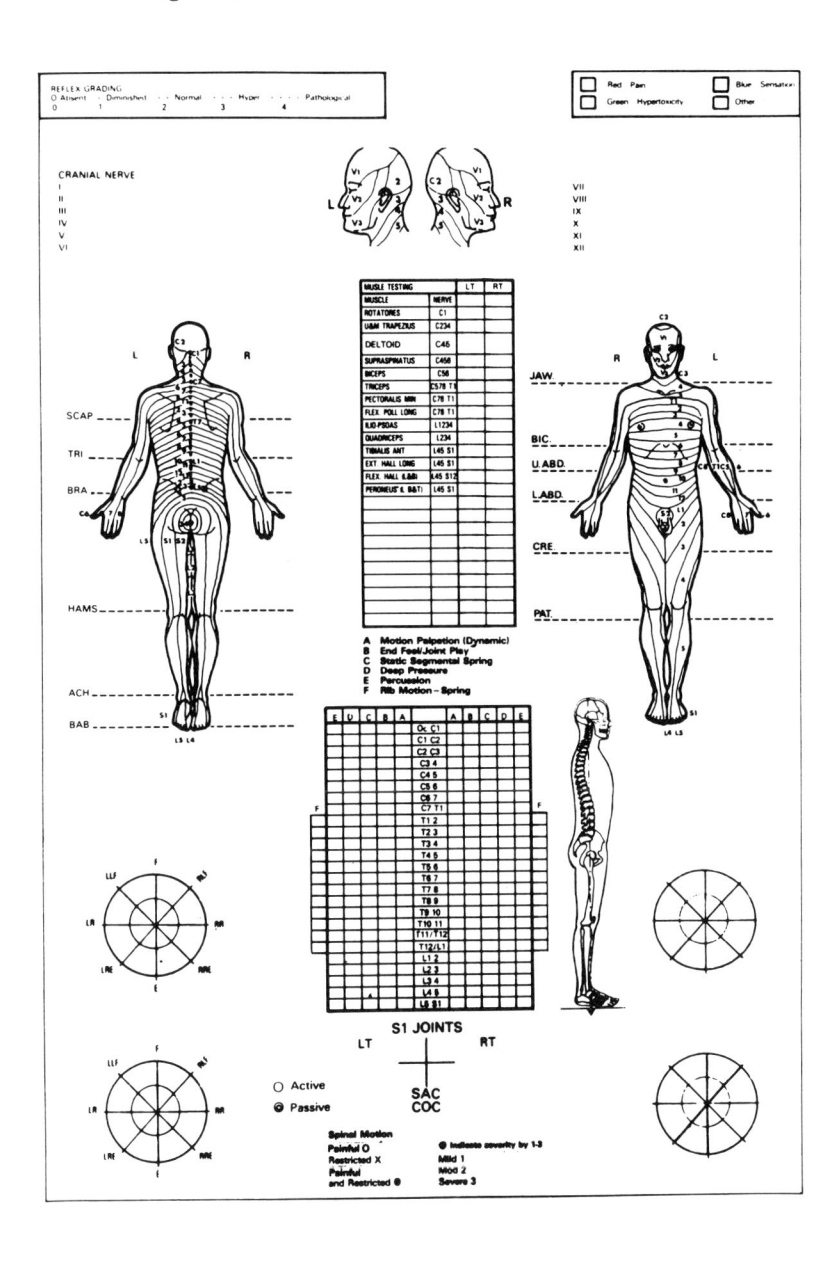

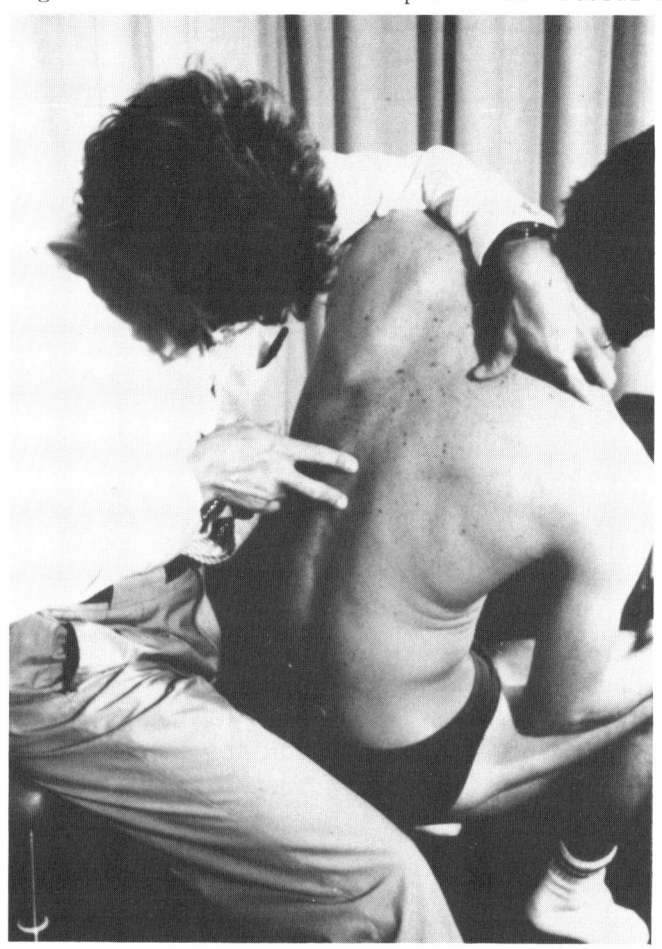

Figure 4. Active Motion Palpation in Lateral Bending.

Figure 5. Normal Joint Range of Motion in a Single Plane (After Sandoz 1976).

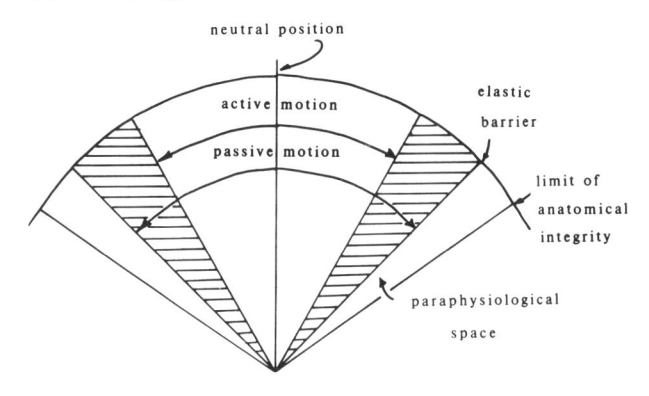

Figure 6. Dynamic Motion Palpation in Relation to Normal Joint Motion.

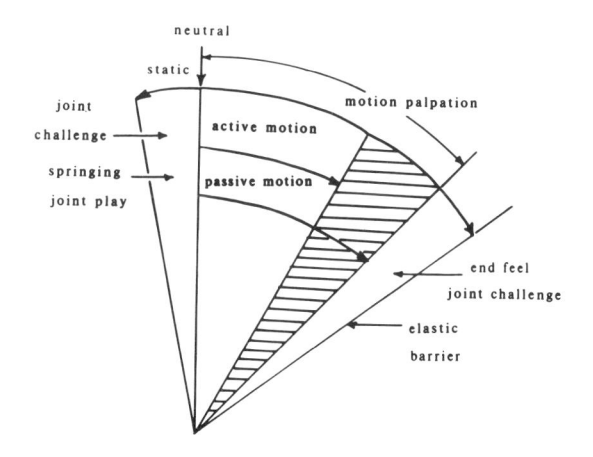

etiological factors of MSD can be forthright to ensure that proper therapeutic intervention and management is the order of the day.

REFERENCES

Andersson, G.B., 1981, Spine, Vol. 6, No. 1 January/February 53-60.

Andersson, G.B., 1981, Spine, Vol. 6, No. 1 January/February 52.

Andersson, G.B., 1985. In Emperical approaches to the validation of Spinal Manipulation, 1st edn, edited by A. A. Buerger & P. Greenman (Charles C. Thomas) 53-70.

Breig, A. & Troup, J.D.G., 1979, Spine, Vol. 4, No. 3, May 242-250.

Brunarski, D.J., 1982, Journal of Manipulative and Physiological Therapeutics, Vol. 5, No. 4 December, 155.

Burton, K., Thompson, J., 1986, Editorials, Clinical Biomechanics, 1, 1-2.

Burton, K., 1986, Clinical Biomechanics, 1, 20-26.

Burton, K., 1986, Meeting Reports - Spinal Mechanics Seminar, St. Aiden's College, University of Durham, April 18-19, 1986 Clinical Biomechanics, 1, 171-173.

Cassidy, J.D., 1976, Journal of the Canadian Chiropractic Association, July, 13-16.

Cassidy, J.D. & Potter, G., 1979, Journal of Manipulative and Physiological Therapeutics, Vol. 2, No. 3, September 151-158.

Cassidy, J.D., Kirkaldy-Willis, W.H. & McGregor, M., 1985 In Emperical approaches to the Validation of Spinal Manipulation, 1st edn, edited by A. A. Buerger, A. & P. Greenman (Charles C. Thomas) 119-148.

Diakow, P.R.P. & Cassidy, J.D., 1984, Journal of Manipulative and Physiological Therapeutics, Vol. 7, No. 2, June 85-88.

Farfan, H.F., 1973, Mechanical disorders of the Low Back, (Lea & Febiger).

Feinstein, B., 1977. In Approaches to the validation of Manipulation Therapy. Edited by A. A. Buerger & J. Tobis (Charles C. Thomas) 139-174.

Fligg, B., 1984, Journal of the Canadian Chiropractic Association, Vol. 28, No. 3, September 331.

Fligg, B., 1985, Journal of the Canadian Chiropractic Association, Vol. 29, No. 3, September 152-153.

Gillet, H., 1960. Annals of the Swiss Chiropractic Association, 1, 30-33.

Gillet, H. & Liekens, M.E., 1981. Belgium Research Chiropractic Notes, 11th edn (Motion Palpation Inst.).

Gitelman, R., 1975. In The Research Status of Spinal Manipulative Therapy, edited by M. Golostein (Nincds Monograph No. 15) Bethesda MD, Dhew, 277-285.
Gitelman, R., Grice, A. & Vernon, H., C.M.C.C. Orthopaedics and Kinesiology Notes, 1978-1980, Unpublished.
Gitelman, R., 1980. In Modern Developments in the Principles and Practice of Chiropractic, 1st edn, edited by S. Haldeman (Appleton-Century-Crofts) 297-330.
Greenman, P., 1985. In Empirical Approaches to the validation of Spinal Manipulation, 1st edn, edited by A. A. Buerger & P. Greenman (Charles C. Thomas) 87-105.
Grice, A.S., 1979. Journal of Manipulative and Physiological Therapeutics, Vol. 2, No. 1, March 26-34.
Grice, A., 1980. In Modern Developments in the Principles and Practice of Chiropractic, 1st edn, edited by S. Haldeman (Appleton-Century-Crofts), 331-358.
Hackett, G., 1958. Ligament and Tendon Relaxation Treated by Prolotherapy, 3rd edn (Charles C. Thomas)
Hoppenfeld, S., 1976. Physical Examination of the Spine and Extremities (Appleton-Century-Crofts).
Kelsey, J.L., White A.A., Pastides, H. & Bisbee, G., 1979, The Journal of Bone and Joint Surgery, American Volume, Vol. 61-A, No. 7, DLT, 959-963.
Kelsey, J.L., 1982. In American Academy of Orthopaedic Surgeons Symposium on Idiopathic Low Back Pain, edited by A. A. White and S. L. Gordon (C.V. Mosby Co. Toronto) 5-8.
Kirkaldy-Willis, W.H. & Hill, R.J., 1979, Spine, Vol. 4, No. 2 March/April, 102-109.
Kirkaldy-Willis, W.H. & Cassidy, J.D., 1985. Canadian Family Physician, Vol. 31, March.
Kirkaldy-Willis, W.H., 1985, Spine, Vol. 10, No. 3, 254.
Lee, P., Helewa, A., Smythe, H. Bombardier, C. & Goldsmith, C., 1985. The Journal of Rheumatology, 12:6, 1169-1173.
Maigne, R., 1972, Orthopaedic Medicine - A new Approach to Vertebral Manipulations. 2nd printing (Charles C. Thomas).
Meal, G., 1977. Bulletin of the European Chiropractic Union, 25 (2), 46-53.
Mennel, J.McM., 1964, Joint Pain Diagnosis and Treatment using Manipulative Techniques, 1st edn (Little, Brown and Company).
Mooney, V. & Robertson, J., 1976. Clinical Orthopaedics 155, 149-156.
Nachemson, A., 1976. Spine, Vol. 1, No. 1 March, 59-67.
O'Brien, J.P., 1984. In Textbook of Pain, edited by P. R. Wall & R. Melzack (Churchill Livingston).

Pearcy, M., 1986. *Clinical Biomechanics*, 1, 44-51.
Sandoz, R., 1976, *Annals of Swiss Chiropractic Association* 6, 91-141.
Terret, A., 1982. *A Method of Examining Low Back*. Preliminary Publication, Department of Diagnostic Sciences.
Troup, J.D.G., Martin, S.W., Lloyd, D.C., 1981. A Prospective Study, *Spine*, Vol. 6, No. 1 January/February 61-65.
Troup, J.D.G., 1986, *Clinical Biomechanics*, 1:31-43.
Valkenburg, H.A. & Haanen, H., 1982. In *American Academy of Orthopaedic Surgeons Symposium on Idiopathic Low Back Pain*, edited by A. A. White and S. L. Gordon (C. V. Mosby Co. Toronto), 9-22.
West, H.G. Jnr., 1980. In *Modern Developments of the Principles and Practice of Chiropractic*, 1st edn, edited by E. S. Haldeman (Appleton-Century-Crofts), 269-296.
White, A.A. & Gordon, S.L., 1982. *Spine*, Vol. 7, No. 2 141
White, A.A., 1982. In *American Academy of Orthopaedic Surgeons Symposium on Idiopathic Low Back Pain*, edited by A. A. White & S. L. Gordon (C.V. Mosby Co. Toronto) 1-2.

COMPARATIVE ANALYSIS OF ELECTRICAL STIMULATION AND EXERCISES TO INCREASE TRUNK MUSCLE STRENGTH AND ENDURANCE

Neil Kahanovitz, M.D., Margareta Nordin, Ph.D., Kathy Viola, RPT, Santiago Yabut, M.D., Mohamad Parnianpour, M.S., and Mike Mulvihill, Dr. PH +

The Back Center and Occupational and Industrial Orthopaedic Center (OIOC), Hospital for Joint Diseases Orthopaedic Institute, 301 East 17th Street, New York, New York, 10003, and +the Department of Community Medicine, Mount Sinai School of Medicine, 1 Gustave Levy Place, New York, New York 10029, U.S.A.

INTRODUCTION

Muscle strength as a possible factor in the etiology of low back pain has received a great deal of attention (Bergquist-Ullman & Larsson 1977). It is, therefore, widely accepted that exercises play an important role in the treatment and prevention of low back pain. The goal of most rehabilitative programs is aimed at improving the trunk strength and endurance of the low back pain patient. Electrical stimulation has been shown to be effective in increasing the strength of the muscles of the lower extremities (Currier et al. 1979, Currier & Mann 1983, Eriksson et al. 1981, Gould et al. 1982, Halbach & Straus 1980, Laughman et al. 1983, McMiken et al. 1983, Romero et al. 1980) but to our knowledge, its effect on trunk muscle strength has not been documented.

The use of electrical stimulation in the lower back has been used predominantly as a pain reduction modality (Melzack et al. 1983, Rutkowski et al. 1980). Electrical stimulation used to improve trunk muscle strength and endurance has not previously been reported.

This prospective controlled study was based on the hypothesis that a strong back is associated with a decreased incidence of low back pain. Therefore, the study was designed to determine whether an exercise or electrical stimulation program was equally effective in increasing isometric/isokinetic strength and endurance of the trunk musculature. The study was also devised to determine if exercise or electrical stimulation was quantifiably superior in increasing the various trunk strength parameters.

MATERIALS AND METHODS

One-hundred-and-seventeen normal females ranging in age from 18-48 (with an average of 28.2 years) participated as volunteers in this study. None of the participants had a recent (>3 months) history of low back pain, and all were examined by a physician. The subjects underwent a test battery (Nordin et al. in press) which consisted of Cybex II (2100 Smithtown Avenue, Ronkonkoma, N.Y. 11779 USA) isometric and isokinetic strength testing of the abdominal and back muscles, Natick standing pull tests (USA Medical Research Institute, Natick, Massachusetts 02741 USA) (Knapik et al. 1981) and the Sorensen endurance test (Biering-Sorensen 1984).

The order of test trials was randomized except for the Sorensen test which was always performed last. Each isometric test and each isokinetic test were performed three times. The mean value of each peak amplitude over the three trials was computed. Isometric tests were performed in a prone and supine position. Isokinetic tests were performed at 30 degrees per second and 60 degrees per second in a sitting posture.

The Natick tests were performed in two ways: - in an upright position with the handle at the height of the axilla of the subject and - with flexed back and bent knees and the handle 38 cm from the floor. Each lift was performed three times with a five second sampling time for each lift. Mean values for the average and maximum force were computed for each trial. Between each test trial of the test battery a period of one minute's rest was given to avoid fatigue.

The Sorensen endurance test was performed in the prone position with the subject firmly strapped to the table over the pelvis, thigh, and lower leg. The subjects were asked to maintain the upper body in the horizontal position for as long as possible, not exceeding a five minute time limit. The test was discontinued when horizontal alignment was no longer maintained. Only one attempt was allowed.

Subjects were randomly assigned to either two types of electrical stimulation (ES1 & ES2), exercise (E), or to a control group (C) (Table 1). The electrical stimulation groups and the exercise group underwent twenty training sessions (five days a week for four weeks), each of which lasted for thirty minutes. The subjects were allowed to miss ten percent of the training sessions before they were excluded from the study. The controls did not receive any intervention.

TABLE 1. CHARACTERISTICS OF SUBJECTS
MEAN VALUES (STANDARD DEVIATIONS) IN AGE, HEIGHT, WEIGHT OF TREATMENT GROUPS

	Group E (n = 22)	Group ES1 (n = 30)	Group ES2 (n = 29)	Group C (n = 18)
Mean Age (years)	27.1 (6.1)	29.5 (6.4)	29.1 (8.2)	30.1 (5.0)
Mean Height (m)	1.6 (8.6)	1.6 (14.3)	1.6 (9.3)	1.6 (6.4)
Mean Weight (kg)	57.6 (8.1)	57.6 (8.1)	57.8 (7.0)	56.6 (8.6)

The electrical stimulation devices used were the Respond,TM, Quadriflex Model 3109(ES1) (Medtronic: 7000 Central Avenue N.E., Minneapolis, Minnesota 55440 USA) and the Soken (ES2) (Rehab Medical Specialties: 1910 Silver Street, Garland, Texas 75042 USA) (Figure 1A). Electrical stimulation was administered in the prone position. Electrodes were placed at L2-L4 levels over the erector spinae muscle bulks (Figure 1B). The intensity of the electrical stimulation was set at the maximum the subject could tolerate for a period of twenty minutes.with an intermittant stimulation. Subjects were given additional five minute warm-up and cool-down periods at lower intensities.

216 Musculoskeletal disorders at work

Figure 1A. Electrical stimulation parameters for the two devices used in the study.

LOW FREQUENCY ELECTRICAL STIMULATION DEVICE (ES1)

MEDIUM FREQUENCY ELECTRICAL STIMULATION DEVICE (ES2)

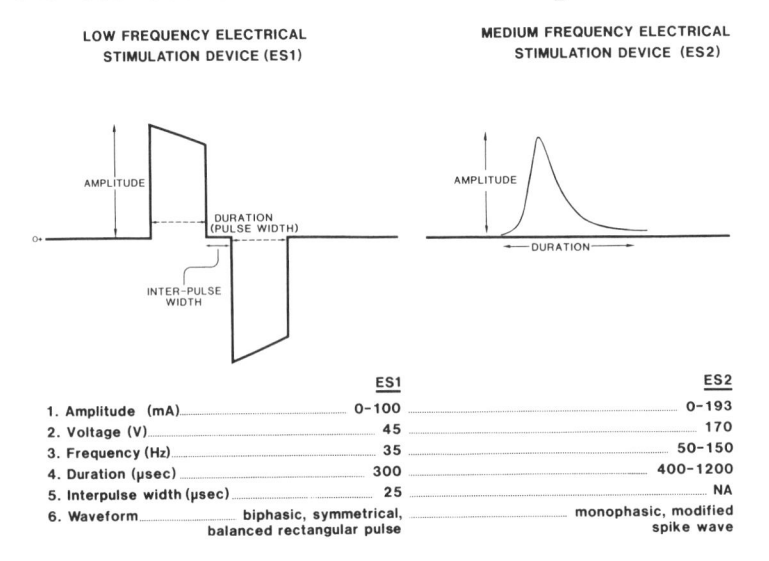

	ES1	ES2
1. Amplitude (mA)	0-100	0-193
2. Voltage (V)	45	170
3. Frequency (Hz)	35	50-150
4. Duration (μsec)	300	400-1200
5. Interpulse width (μsec)	25	NA
6. Waveform	biphasic, symmetrical, balanced rectangular pulse	monophasic, modified spike wave

Figure 1B. Electrode placement during stimulation.

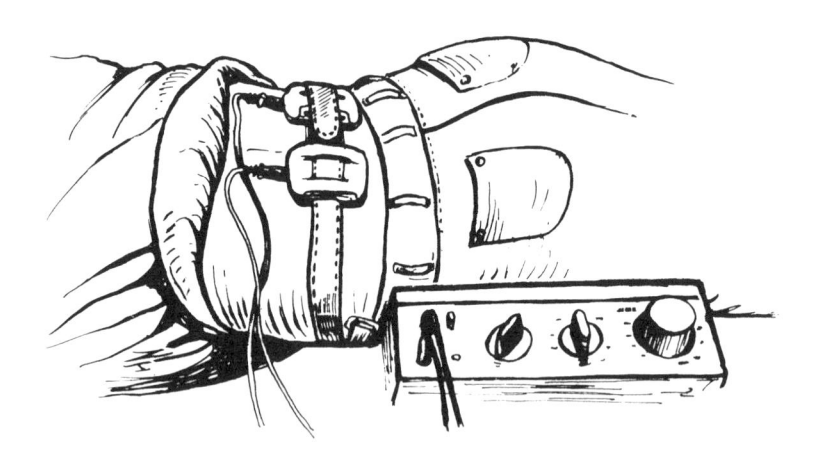

The subjects in the exercise group had a warm-up and cool-down period consisting of five minutes of stretching, followed by a program of twenty minutes of back exercises. These consisted of prone trunk extension exercises, prone leg lifts, prone arm lifts and a combination of "all fours" arms- and -leg-lifts.

Following the training period 99 subjects repeated the test battery in the same randomized order as the pretest and during the same time of the day as their initial testing. The test personnel were not aware of the actual grouping of the subjects.

STATISTICAL ANALYSIS

The four groups (ES1, ES2, E and C) were evaluated for compatability at $p < .05$ level by a one-way analysis of variance for all parameters studied, including demographic and strength variables. Since strength and endurance parameters after the intervention area function of the initial strength of the individual (baseline values), the analysis focused on changes in strength and endurance following the intervention. This was done by subtracting the pre-intervention strength measures from the post-intervention strength levels. Mean change was then computed for each of the study groups. In those instances in which a statistical significance was demonstrated, a students t-test was performed for each of the treatment groups compared to the controls as well as between the three treatment groups. For this study a statistical significance level of $p < .05$ was chosen for the t-test.

RESULTS

The results of this study show a consistent pattern. Subjects undergoing electrical stimulation (ES1 & ES2) and the exercise program (E), increased significantly in isokinetic strength ($p < .05$). The subjects undergoing muscle stimulation also increased significantly in endurance ($p < .008$) compared to the control and exercise groups. For the isometric tests, no significant increase in strength occurred for the exercise group and both ES groups. However, compared to the C-group all subjects receiving either electrical stimulation or exercises showed an increase in strength in isometric extension.

Electrical stimulation with low frequency (ES1) and exercises (E) gave a similar significant increase in most measured strength parameters in comparison with the control group (C). These results did not occur for stimulation with medium high frequency (ES2).

DISCUSSION

The effect of electrical stimulation on back muscle strength and endurance has not previously been documented to our knowledge. This study suggests that with low frequency electrical stimulation, isokinetic strength and endurance may be significantly increased. This was not true, however, for medium frequency stimulation.

Electrical stimulation, a passive modality of muscle strengthening, may be better tolerated than exercise for a patient with acute or sub-acute low back pain. Electrical stimulation also has the added advantage of providing an anaesthetic effect from the stimulation which may also decrease pain while treatment is being administered. It must be recognized that selective training with electrical stimulation or exercise, or a combination of both, can be used to obtain optimal clinical results. Electrical stimulation may therefore become a valuable treatment modality for patients with acute and sub-acute back pain before beginning an exercise conditioning program.

REFERENCES

Bergquist-Ullman, M., Larsson, U., 1977, Acute low back pain in industry: A controlled prospective study with special reference to therapy and vocational factors. Acta Orthopedica Scandinavica. (Suppl. 170).

Biering-Sorensen, F., 1984, Physical measurements as risk indicators for low back trouble over a one year period. Spine, 9, 106.

Currier, D.P., Lehman, J., Lightfoot, P., 1979, Electrical stimulation in exercise of the quadriceps femoris muscle. Physical Therapy, 59, 1508.

Currier, D.P., Mann, R., 1983, Muscular strength development by electrical stimulation in healthy individuals. Physical Therapy, 63, 915.

Eriksson, E., Haggmark, T., Kiessling, K.H., Karlsson, J., 1981, Effect of electrical stimulation on human skeleton muscle. International Journal of Sports Medicine, 2, 18.

Gould, N., Donnermeyer, D., Pope, M., Ashikaga, T., 1982, Transcutaneous muscle stimulation as a method to retard disuse atrophy. Clinical Orthopaedics, 164, 215.

Halbach, J.W., Straus, D., 1980, Comparison of electro-myo stimulation to isokinetic training in increasing power of the knee extensor mechanism. Journal of Orthopaedics Sports Physical Therapy, 2, 20.

Knapik, J.J., Vogel, J.A., Wright, J.E., 1981, Measurement of isometric strength in an upright pull at 38 cm. USA Medical Research Institute of Environmental Medicine, (Natick, Massachusetts) Report Number T 3/81.

Laughman, R.K., Youdas, J.W., Garrett, T.R., Chao, E.Y.S., 1983, Strength changes in the normal quadriceps femoris as a result of electrical stimulation. Physical Therapy, 63, 494.

McMiken, D.F., Todd-Smith, M., Thompson, C., 1983, Strengthening of human quadriceps muscles by cutaneous electrical stimulation. Scandinavian Journal of Rehabilitative Medicine, 15, 25.

Melzack, R., Vetere, P., Finch, L., 1983, Transcutaneous electrical nerve stimulation for low back pain: A comparison of TENS and massage for pain and range of motion. Physical Therapy, 63, 489.

Nordin, M., Kahanovitz, N., Verderame, R., Parnianpour, M., Yabut, S., Viola, K., Greenidge, N., Normal endurance and trunk muscle strength in 101 adult females. Spine (in press).

Romero, J.A., Sanford, T.L., Schroeder, R.V., Fahey, T.D., 1980, The effects of electrical stimulation of normal quadriceps on strength and girth. Medical Science Sports Exercise, 14, 194.

Rutkowski, B., Neidzialkowska, T., Otto, J., 1977, Electrical stimulation in chronic low-back pain. British Journal of Anaesthesiology, 49, 629.

THE LOW-BACK PAIN PREVAILING AMONG
THE FREIGHT-CONTAINER TRACTOR DRIVERS IN JAPAN

M. NAKATA, K. NISHIYAMA and S. WATANABE

Department of Preventive Medicine,
Shiga University of Medical Science,
Seta, Tsukinowa-cho, Otsu, 520-21 Japan

INTRODUCTION

The containerization of liner freight has been rapidly developing in Japan since 1967, and it amounted to more than two thirds of the export and import freight in the early 1980s. About 5,800 exclusive semi-trailer tractors are active now for domestic ground transport with the 20 or 40 foot-long containers. The only task of tractor drivers is driving, being free from handling of the freight, but many of them complain of low-back pain (LBP).

To make clear the causal factors of this LBP, the vibration measurement of the seat, ergonomical check of the tractors, survey on the working hours and medical examination were carried out.

METHODS

1. Vibration measurements were made on 9 kinds of popularly-used freight-container tractors with or without freight on selected public roads (80km). One heavy duty truck was also measured at the same conditions as a reference. The pick-up was set under the driver's buttocks on the seat.

The time-weighted mean of vibration level was measured according to the weighting method of ISO 2631, and the allowable exposure time was then obtained from the fatigue-decreased proficiency boundary (FDP) and exposure limit (EL) in ISO 2631.

2. Survey on the working hours and distance travelled were

Table. Mean vibration level of the vehicles (dB) and its evaluation by fatigue-decreased proficiency boundary (FDP) and exposure limit (EL) of ISO 2631.

Tractor		Time required (min)	Mean vibration level(dB)* and direction	Allowable exposure time (min)	
				FDP	EL
A-old:	U	73	93.1 (X)	170	470
	L	81	97.1 (X)	82	240
A-imp+:	U	79	94.0 (X)	150	410
	L	77	95.4 (X)	110	330
A-new:	U	76	93.8 (X)	150	420
	L	73	95.4 (X)	110	330
A-new:	U	66	96.2 (X)	98	280
(40ft)	L	75	94.8 (X)	130	360
B-old:	U	60	96.4 (X)	94	270
	L	71	96.4 (X)	94	270
B-new:	U	70	93.4 (X)	170	450
	L	81	94.7 (X)	130	360
C-old:	U	67	96.2 (X)	98	280
	L	75	96.0 (X)	100	290
C-new:	U	76	94.8 (X)	130	360
	L	78	95.5 (X)	110	320
D-old:	U	63	97.3 (X)	78	230
	L	67	98.0 (X)	68	210
D-new:	U	66	94.4 (X)	140	380
	L	64	97.4 (Z)	140	390
Mean :	U	70	95.0 (X)	120	350
	L	75**	95.5** (Z)	100**	290**
Truck:	U	68	95.7 (Z)	190	480<
	L	62	95.0 (Z)	220	480<

U : Unloaded condition.
L : Loaded condition.
* : Mean vibration level and its direction which make the allowable exposure time the shortest.
** : Calculated value from nine X directions.
\+ : Improved A-old model.

calculated from the daily working records of a month of 240 drivers. A more precise time-study was carried out on 6 drivers during 7 days to calculate the mean speed of the tractors in various routes.

From these two studies, the daily vibration exposure time was estimated on each labour day of each driver, which came to a total of 5,163 days.

3. Ergonomical evaluation of the freight-container tractors was made using an ergonomical checklist consisting of 130 items on the matters of getting in and out of the cabin, space size of the cabin, driver's seat, steering wheel, pedals, levers, visual range from the cabin, noise, vibration, condition of the air, some operations performed outside the cabin, etc. The checklist was filled in by 549 drivers.

4. Medical examination, primarily composed of orthopedic examinations and questioning on health conditions, was performed on 231 drivers whose mean age was 38.6 yrs (87% in 30-40 yrs) and whose experience as a tractor driver was 8.8+4.5 yrs on an average.

RESULTS

1. The vibration of the tractor seat was at a high level in the X direction, equal to or exceeding that in the Z direction, which is dominant in ordinary vehicles. So, the direction in which the allowable exposure time from the point of view of FDP and EL was the shortest was the X direction in all cases except one (see Table).

The allowable exposure time of each tractor was considerably shorter than that of the heavy duty truck.

2. In more than 90% of the 5,163 work-days, the driving hours (estimated vibration exposure time) exceeded the allowable exposure time from the viewpoint of FDP, and in more than 30% exceeded the allowable exposure time from that of EL.

3. The ergonomical check on the tractors revealed various problems, among which there were many concerned with muscle fatigue, for instance, difficulties in getting in and out of the cabin, narrow foot space of the cabin, unfitness of the driver's seat to the driver's body, difficulties in using pedals and gearshift, steering wheel

Figure 1. Positive rate of tenderness test on various muscles of the right side of body. (The results on the left side is similar to this except thenar muscles.) Symbols; see Figure 2.

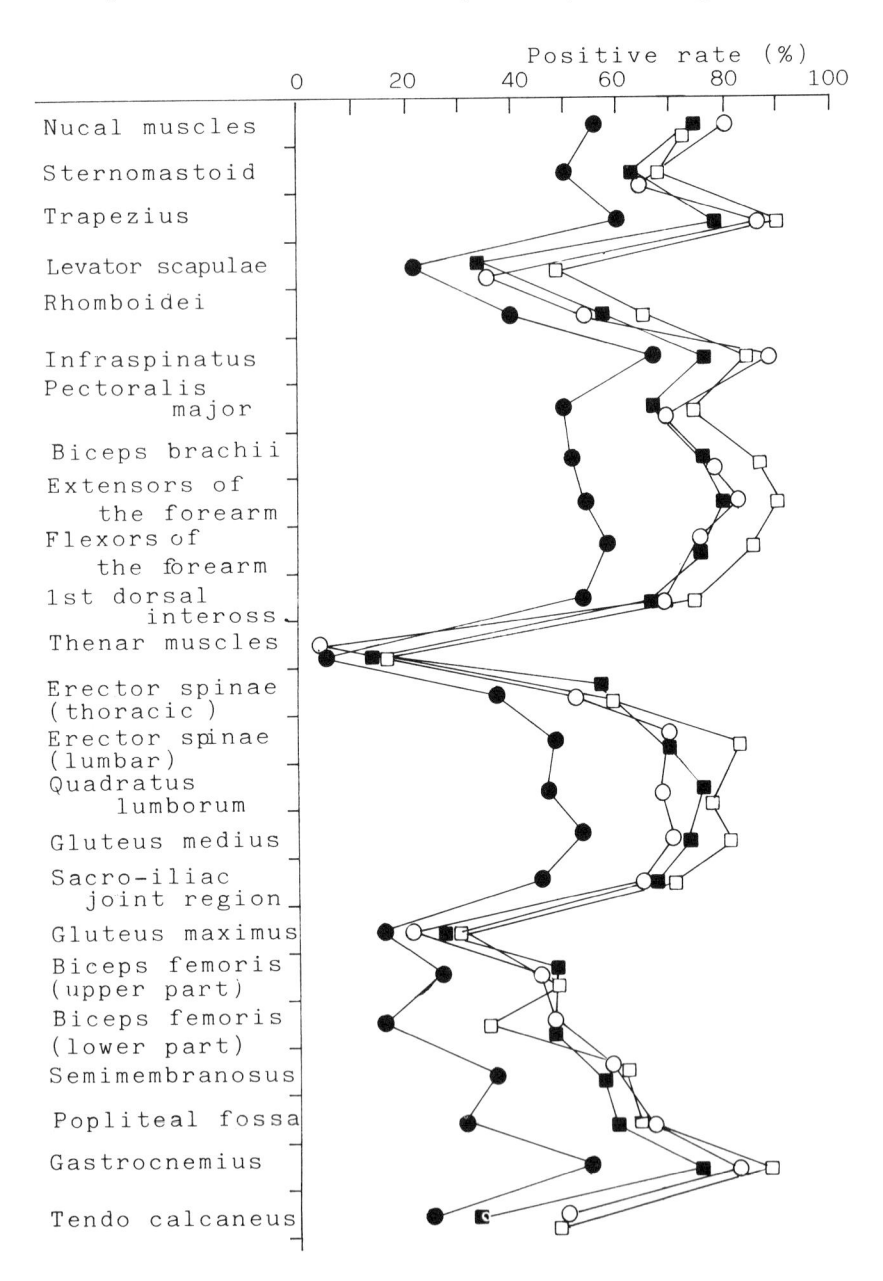

Figure 2. Positive rate of tenderness and/or percussion-pain test on the spinous processes by the grade of low-back complaints.

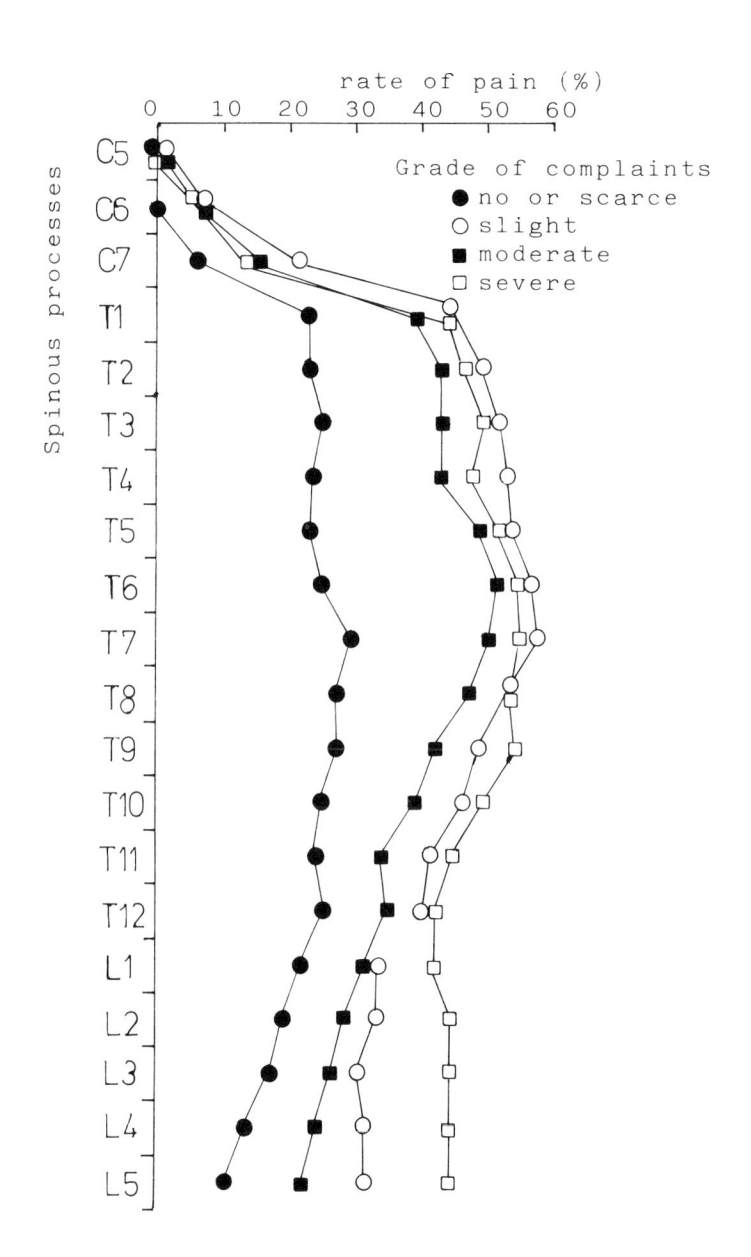

being hard to turn, the necessity of frequently bracing the legs to support the body on severe vibration or shock, etc. All of these were pointed out by more than half of the drivers.

4. Prevailing complaints were dullness or stiffness of the shoulders in 71%, dullness of the neck in 69%, dullness of the low-back in 62%, LBP in 42%, dullness of the lower limbs in 39% and dullness of the back in 36%.

The rates of complaints of dullness or pain of neck, back, or lower limbs, and disturbance of daily activity were associated with the grade of LBP evaluated from the subjective symptoms.

Orthopedic examination revealed an increased tonus or fatigue sign of muscles of the body trunk and limbs, i.e., a high positive rate of tenderness (see Figure 1), percussion pain on the spinous processes (see Figure 2), and poor results in the tests on back and abdominal muscle strength and durability.

These findings were seen more frequently in the group with subjective symptoms, but also among the group without symptoms in some degree, suggesting the existence of latent LBP cases.

CONCLUSIONS

From these findings, the characteristic of the LBP prevailing among the freight-container tractor drivers seems to originate in the accumulated or chronic fatigue mainly extending over a wide area of the erector spinae.

Moreover, that fatigue was recognized as that derived from daily exposure to the severe vibration of the tractor for a long time and ergonomically problematic conditions of the tractor which demand strong muscle power or continuous static tension of muscles.

REFERENCES

International Organization for Standardization, 1978, Guide for the evaluation of human exposure to whole-body vibration, 2nd edn (ISO 2631-1978 (E)).
Nakata, M. & Nishiyama, K., 1986, Labor of freight-container tractor drivers and low-back pain: correlation with whole-body vibration exposure. Japanese Journal of Industrial Health, 28, p341-351.

INTRODUCTION OF STANDING AIDS IN THE FURNITURE INDUSTRY

Irene NIJBOER & Jan DUL

TNO-Institute of Preventive Health Care,
P.O. Box 124,
NL-2300 AC Leiden, The Netherlands

ABSTRACT

The aim of this study is to stimulate the use of standing aids at the upholstering workplace in the Dutch furniture industry. A simple method is developed to analyse the attitude of management concerning these aids. The results show that misunderstandings about disadvantages of the use of standing aids - and not finances - are the major reasons for not buying standing aids. Relevant information on these items may stimulate the introduction of standing aids at the workplace.

INTRODUCTION

Ergonomists often recommend the use of technical aids to reduce physical load during work. Examples of such aids are lifting aids for nurses (Kilbom et al., 1985), tiltable chairs in offices (Bendix, 1986) and standing aids in industry (Windberg, et al., 1982). However, a common problem is that companies often hesitate to invest in even simple and inexpensive aids. One way of stimulating this investment is to give proper information to the management.

As a result of an ergonomic survey on the quality of working conditions in the Dutch furniture industry, the introduction of standing aids at several workplaces requiring prolonged standing was recommended (Dul, 1985). A standing aid has a forward sloping seat on which a person leans (see Figure 1b). The seat is higher than in a normal chair. A standing aid allows alterations in one's posture between standing and "semi-sitting" (Andersson, 1986). At present several types of standing aids are commercially available. From our survey it has appeared that standing

228 Musculoskeletal disorders at work

aids are particularly useful at the upholstering workplace. This type of work consists of fixing textile or leather seat covers on wooden frames, and it is normally done in a standing posture.

A pilot study was started to find out about which items managers should be informed to stimulate the introduction of standing aids at the upholstering workplace in the furniture industry. The most suitable commercially available aid was selected and was tested at the workplace. The possible reasons for not buying the aids were analysed and compared with the results of the test at the workplace.

METHODS
Description of workplace

In the upholstering workplace chairs and other sitting furniture are being upholstered. Figure 1 shows a typical workplace.

Figure 1. The upholstering workplace in the furniture industry (a. without using standing aid. b. using standing aid).

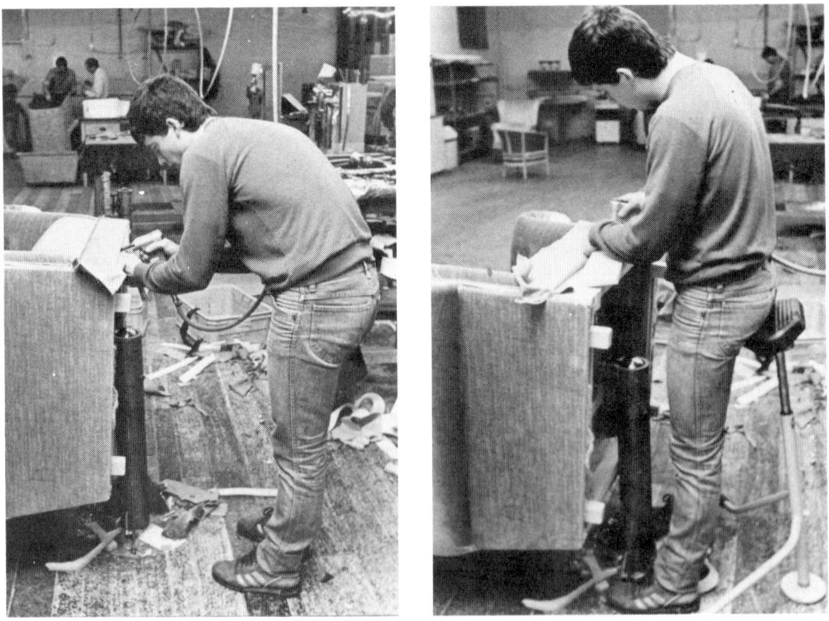

The worker stands for long periods of time on one side of the pillar, which holds the furniture, moves around it, and reaches towards the furniture. In one hand he holds a stapler. At this workplace, standing aids can be used since there is enough room for the worker and the standing aid and if necessary, the aid can easily be put aside. Furthermore, the workplace meets the requirements that the risk of slipping is minimal (no dirt on the floor, sufficient friction between floor and standing aid), and that there are no dangerous machines near by (Windberg et al., 1982).

Selection of standing aids

Table 1. shows six types of standing aids which are commercially available in the Netherlands (prices range from $ 50 to $ 200). Each aid was evaluated with respect to several ergonomical and safety aspects (Van Buchem, 1973; Windberg et al., 1982).

Table 1. Characteristics and evaluation of six commercially available standing aids.

Aspects	standing aid [1]					
	1	2	3	4	5	6
height range (cm)	65-83	65-90	65-90	65-55	68-81	47-86
forward slope (degrees)	10-15	30	10[2]	0-20	5	5
freedom of body movements[3]	++	±	±	+	+	±
safety[3]	±	−	+	+	+	−

1) detailed information can be obtained from the authors.
2) backward slope.
3) − is bad; ± is moderate; + is good; ++ is very good.

It turns out that all aids have acceptable height range. The forward slope of the seat is sufficiently large in only three aids (1, 2 and 4). Because the freedom of body movement is an important aspect in upholstering, standing aid no 1 was selected for this type of work (see Figure 2).

Figure 2. The selected standing aid for the upholstering workplace (number 1 in table 1).

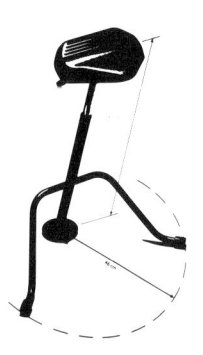

Test at the workplace

The selected aid was introduced at two upholstering workplaces and a detailed instruction was given to the workers. After four weeks several employees were interviewed about their experiences.

It turned out that the worker must decide himself for which activities the aid is appropriate. The aid is particularly useful during upholstering of small pieces of furniture. The aid can be used for about 15% of the working time (several periods of at least 3 minutes). According to experts (e.g. Van Buchem, 1973), this is sufficient to have positive effects. Although the period of time using the aid was short, employees reported that working with standing aids is comfortable, and it appears that the production rate is not negatively effected.

Determinants of the behaviour of managers

To find out about which items managers should be informed, it is necessary to know the determinants of the behaviour of management towards these aids. This was measured by interviewing managers of nine Dutch furniture factories. (The inverviews were semi-structured.) Based on a social psychological model of behaviour (De Vries & Kok, 1986) we distinguished three categories of determinants of this behaviour:
1. the financial limitations;
2. the perceived opinion of colleagues within the company;
3. the expected advantages and disadvantages of the use of standing aids.

RESULTS

Most of the interviewed managers knew about the existance of standing aids. However, none of them had purchased a standing aid. Table 2 shows some relevant results of the interviews.

Table 2. most mentioned responses of managers about standing aids (n=9).

category	type of response	number of responses (%)
1 Financial limitations	investment possible	9 (100%)
2 Perceived opinion of colleagues	colleagues positive	4 (44%)
	don't know the opinion of colleagues	2 (22%)
	no colleagues involved	2 (22%)
	colleagues negative	1 (11%)
3a Expected advantages	less fatigue	6 (67%)
	reduction of low back pain	4 (44%)
	increased motivation	4 (44%)
3b Expected disadvantages	limited freedom of body movement	6 (67%)
	only short period of time useful	4 (44%)

From the responses of managers it can be observed that finances (category 1) are not the reasons of not buying the aids. All interviewed persons reported that the investments are possible. Furthermore almost no one noticed a negative opinion of colleagues within the company towards standing aids (category 2). So, this aspect also does not appear to be a reason of not buying the aids. The expected advantages (category 3a) are very positive, and cannot be a reason of not bying the aids as well. The expected disadvantage (category 3b) 'limited freedom of body movement' means that managers think that the task cannot be done while using a standing aid. The disadvantage 'only a short period of time useful' means that managers think that the aid will not have positive effect because of the short period of time that it can be used. These expected disadvantages can be the reasons of not buying the aids.

These mentioned disadvantages appear to be misunderstandings. One of the mentioned disadvantages: (limited freedom of body movement), does not correspond with our findings during the testing at the workplace. The other disadvantage mentioned (only short period of time useful) is correct, but the period appeared to be sufficient to have positive effects (see section Methods).

To stimulate the introduction of standing aids, the information for management should take away these misunderstandings and therefore stress the following aspects:
- the employee using the selected aid has sufficient freedom of body movement;
- although the period of time the aid can be used may be short, it is sufficient to obtain a positive result.

It appears to us that the expected advantages (category 3a) may be too optimistic. Less fatigue particularly in the legs, may be realistic, but reduction of low back pain and increase of motivation has not yet been demonstrated.

DISCUSSION AND CONCLUSIONS

The purpose of this study was to get an indication of the type of information that could stimulate the introduction of standing aids in the furniture industry. For this purpose we developed a simple interview method, based upon a social psychological model.

The results of the study show that the method is useful and can indeed give some indications about relevant information for managers. However, because only a small number of semi-structured interviews were taken, strict conclusions cannot be drawn.

The starting point of this study was that the use of a standing aid during prolonged standing improves the quality of working conditions. More research is needed to determine the effects of standing aids on workload and health.

The presented study deals with the necessary information for managers in the furniture industry. To stimulate the actual use of standing aids the users, the employees, should be informed. In a parallel study, not reported here, behaviour determinants of employees are analysed, to get an indication about the type of information that could stimulate the proper use of standing aids at the workplace.

ACKNOWLEDGEMENTS

This study was initiated by the "Stichting Sectorbeleid Meubelindustrie" (a foundation with representatives of employers and employees in the Dutch furniture industry) and financially supported by the Dutch Ministry of Social Affairs and Employment. Mrs. Edith Wortel and Mr. Gerjo Kok are thanked for their advice.

REFERENCES

Andersson, G.B.J., 1986, Loads on the spine during sitting. In: The Ergonomics of Working Postures, p. 309-318, Edited by N. Corlett, J. Wilson, I. Manenica (Taylor & Francis), London and Philadelphia.

Bendix, T., 1986, Chair and table adjustments for seated work. In: The Ergonomics of Working Postures, p. 355-362, Edited by N. Corlett, J. Wilson, I. Manenica (Taylor & Francis), London and Philadelphia.

Buchem, P.J.A. van, 1973, The standing Aid as a Solution Between Standing and Sitting MS.-thesis, Delft University of Technology.(in Dutch).

Dul, J., 1985, Working Conditions in the Furniture Industry, Report S-16, Ministry of Social Affairs and Employment, The Hague (In Dutch).

Kilbom, A. Ljundberg, A.S. & Hägg, G., 1985, Lifting and carrying in geriatic care. A comparison between differences in workspace lay out, work organization and use of modern equipment. In: Proceedings of the ninth Congress of the International Ergonomics Association, 2-6 September 1985, Bournebouth, England.

Vries, H. de & G.J. Kok, 1986. From determinants of smoking behaviour to the implications for a prevention programme. Health Education Research No. 1, pg 85-94.

Windberg, H.J., Rademacher, U. & Lange, W., 1982, Stehhilfen am Arbeitsplatz, Möglichkeiten und Grenzen ihres Einsatzes, Forschungsbericht Nr. 322, Bundesanstalt für Arbeitsschutz und Unfall/Forschung, Dortmund, BRD.

CORRELATION BETWEEN DIFFERENT TESTS OF TRUNK STRENGTH

M. Parnianpour, M. Nordin,
U. Moritz, N. Kahanovitz

Occupational & Industrial Orthopaedic Center Hospital for Joint Diseases Orthopaedic and Institute, and Program of Ergonomics and Occupational Biomechanics. New York University 301 East 17th Street, New York, N.Y., 10003, U.S.A.

INTRODUCTION

Epidemiological studies implicate certain mechanical factors for low back injury such as vibration, heavy lifting, strenuous work, bending and twisting in conjunction with lifting, and prolonged constrained posture. Many biomechanical studies have been done to quantify properties of both passive and active components of the spine. Assessment of strength and endurance of back and abdominal muscles, the active elements, are of interest to establish a data base for the normal population and to be used as an objective measure for diagnosis and prognosis of low back patients. In addition, Keyserling et al. (1980) showed that job simulated strength tests can prevent up to one third of work related injuries. Considering that more women enter the work force each year, a data base on strength and endurance of the female population becomes, more necessary. Nicolaisen & Jorgensen (1985) showed that isometric strength per se is of no prognostic value for subsequent development of low back pain. Isometric endurance of the back muscles may prevent first time occurrence of low back trouble in men (Biering-Sorenson 1984). Strength and endurance have been principally measured in isometric and isokinetic modes. Some confusion and controversy exist about the inter-relationship between these modes of testing. This study investigates the inter-correlations between isometric, isokinetic strength and isometric endurance capacity of back muscles.

METHODS

One-hundred-thirty-one normal females participated as volunteers in this study. Their mean (SD) age, weight, height, were 28 (6) years, 58 (9) kilograms, 1.6 (.1) meters respectively. After screening by a physician, all subjects underwent a comprehensive test battery which consisted of isometric and isokinetic strength testing of abdominal and back muscles using a Cybex II Dynamometer (2100 Smithtown Avenue, Ronkonkoma N.Y. 11779,USA), Natick upright pull test (Knapik et al. 1981) and the Sorenson endurance test (Biering-Sorenson 1984). The order of test trials was randomly selected except for the Sorenson test which was performed the last. Isometric back and abdominal muscle strength were measured in prone and supine positions respectively with the axis of rotation at 3 cm below the iliac crest. The isokinetic tests were performed in a sitting position at 30 and 60 degrees per second. The Natick upright pull testswere performed in two different postures: - an upright position with the handle at the level of the axilla and with a straight back and knees, and - with straight a back and bent knees with the handle at 38 cm above the floor. The isometric endurance capacity test was performed in the prone position with the subject firmly strapped to the table. All tests except the endurance test were repeated three times with a one minute rest period between each trial. Mean and standard deviation for all parameters were computed. Correlation coefficients was determined between all parameters using SAS statistical package.

RESULTS

No significant correlation was found between peak torque of isometric abdominal strength test with other parameters. The other isometric test had a very weak correlation ranging from 0.40 to 0.52 (p<.001) amongst themselves, the highest being between the two Natick tests. The Sorenson test and isometric and isokinetic strength parameters had also weak, but significant correlations, ranging from 0.21 to 0.40 (p<.01), the best being with the total energy of isokinetic flexion and extension at 30 degrees/second. The correlation coefficient between isometric and isokinetic strength parameters ranged from 0.28 to 0.52 ($p<.001$), with the highest being between isometric and isokinetic peak torque extension at 30 degrees per second. The strongest correlations were obtained amongst the isokinetic strength parameters ranging from 0.54 to 0.94 ($p<.001$), with the highest being the extension peak torque and the peak torque value at 30 degrees of range of motion for the 60 degrees/second test.

The extension peak torque at this speed occurred at 27 (16) degrees. The correlation coefficient of the same isokinetic strength parameters between two speeds ranged from 0.79 to 0.87 ($p<.001$). The strength parameters were both a function of position and velocity of trunk.

The complete data on strength and endurance and their intercorrelation matrix can be obtain from the authors.

DISCUSSION

The normal data is compared with data previously reported in literature. The isometric mean value of trunk flexor and extensor is lower than those reported by Hause et al. (1980). The isokinetic values are in this study lower than those found by Langrana et al.(1984) which could be due to slight differences in positioning and stabilization. The Natick test results represent a 20% lower values than Knapik et al. (1981) reported for the U.S. Army which is expected because the population in this study were older and drawn from a general population. The isometric endurance of trunk extensors had the highest correlation, ($r=0.41$, $p<.001$), with total energy in extension at both 30 and 60 degrees/seconds. A number of significant correlations exist but too weak to have any predictive power. The unexpected results were that isometric endurance had better correlation with isokinetic parameters than with isometric parameters.

The correlation amongst the isometric tests were low. The isometric results also showed low correlation with isokinetic testing modes. There was no significant correlation amongst the maximum isometric flexion and any isometric or isokinetic parameter. However, there was good correlation amongst the isokinetic parameters.

These results are in complete agreement with Thorstensson & Nilsson (1982) and Ostering et al. (1977). Thorstensson & Nilsson (1982) showed that the strength is function of both movement velocity, body position, and center of rotation. This data further supports the conclusion of Mital & Karwowski (1985) who showed that the use of static strength testing to develop human performance limit for dynamic tasks is fundamentally incorrect since the inertial forces are ignored. Marras et al. (1984) showed that muscles recruitment patterns are drastically different between static and isokinetic movements. In addition, another ignored parameters is the time available to complete a lifting task. Hall (1985) demonstrated that faster lifting significantly increase compressive and shear forces at L5/S1 level and generates higher external moment to be balanced by the muscles and other structure of the back. Strength is a complicated quantity that has to be measured through a number of parameters and based on this study isometric tests cannot substitute isokinetic tests. McNeill et al. (1980) showed equal isometric trunk muscle strength for back patients as for normals. However Langrana et al. (1984) showed significant differences in isokinetic torque curves between patients versus normals thus making dynamic strength assessment indispensable.

CONCLUSION

Strength and endurance data were collected for 131 normal females and the intercorrelation of these parameters of strength were investigated. Poor correlations were found amongst different isometric and isokinetic parameters which explain the need for dynamic assessment of strength and endurance for job preplacement and low back pain predictors.

REFERENCES

Biering-Sorenson, F., 1984, Physical measurements as risk indicator for low-back trouble over a one-year period, Spine, 9, 106.

Hall, S., 1985, Effect of attempted lifting speed on forces and torque exerted on the lumbar spine . Medicine and Science in Sports and Exercise, 15, 440.

Hause, M., Fujiwara, M., Kikuchi, S., 1980, A new method of quantitative measurement of abdominal and back muscle strength. Spine, 5, 143.

Keyserling, W., Herrin, G., Chaffin, D., 1980, Isometric strength testing as a means of controlling medical incidents on strenuous jobs, Journal of Occupational Medicine, 22, 332.

Knapik, J., Vogel, J., Wright, J., 1981, Measurment of the isometric strength in an upright pull at 38 cm. USA Med. Rsch Inst. of Env. Med.,Natick, Massachusetts, Report Number T 3/81.

Langrana, N., Lee, C., Alexander, H., Mayott, C.,1984, Quantitative assessment of back strength using isokinetic testing. Spine, 5, 287.

Marras, W., King, A., Joynt, R., 1984, Measurements of loads on the lumbar spine under isometric and isokinetic conditions, Spine, 9, 176.

McNeill, T., Warwick, D., Andersson, G., Schultz, A., 1980, Trunk strengths in attempted flexion, extension, and lateral bending in healthy subjects and patients with low back disorbers. Spine, 5, 529.

Mital, A., Karwowski, W., 1985, Use of Simulated job dynamic strength (SJDS) in screening workers for Manual lifting tasks. Proceedings of Human Factors Society 29th Annual Meeting, 513.

Nicolaisen, T., Jorgensen, K., 1985, Trunk strength, back muscle endurance and low back trouble, Scandinavian Journal of Rehabilitation Medicine, 17,1985, 121.

Ostering, R., Bates, B., James, S.,1977, Isokinetic and isometric torque relationship, Archives Physical Medicine Rehabilitation, 58, 254.

Thorstensson, A., Nilsson, J., 1982, Trunk Muscle Strength During Constant Velocity Movements. Scandinavian Journal of Rehabilitation Medicine, 14, 61.

DEVELOPMENT OF A PRACTICAL METHOD FOR WORKPLACE REDESIGN TO REDUCE UPPER LIMB STRAIN INJURY

A.J. Pethick, M.H. Mabey and R.J. Graves

Ergonomics Branch, Institute of Occupational Medicine,
c/o British Coal HQ Technical Department,
Stanhope Bretby, Burton-on-Trent, Staffordshire DE15 OQD

SUMMARY
The paper describes the development of a method to quantify upper limb components during on-site assessments of industrial tasks. The methodology is particularly useful in assessing the task elements which may contribute to the occurrence of Upper Limb Strain Injury (ULSI). Task features are quantified in each case so that those needing to be changed, in order to reduce the likelihood of ULSI, can be readily identified. Examples are given which illustrate the practical application of the methodology. It is suggested that such an approach provides more objective data than is normally available to complement professional opinion. This is of importance in improving design in the interim period while research is being carried out into definitive criteria and causal relationships.

INTRODUCTION
The increased concern about musculoskeletal disorders of the hand, wrist and arm - upper limb strain injuries (ULSI) - as a health problem has highlighted the need for some means of reducing the occurrence. Task design has been suggested as the most cost-effective means of minimising ULSI. However, for this approach to be effective, there is a need to evaluate the task components objectively to identify those which exceed criteria of acceptability for forces, posture and repetition. This information is needed to identify those factors causing problems and to assist in setting priorities for redesign. Few examples of either specific or general guidance on the objective evaluation of upper limb task components have been found in the literature. Also, little detail has been

written on how to design jobs and equipment to minimise upper limb musculoskeletal problems.

The paper describes the development of a method, during 1984, to provide objective support for expert opinion. It covers the derivation of "working" criteria and examples of the use of the methodology in assessing problems and assisting in redesign in industry.

To evaluate task elements objectively, it is necessary to measure the angles of limbs, assess forces being applied by the worker, and quantify the number of repetitions of the task elements. This data then needs to be compared with criteria to provide a basis for determining whether there is likely to be a contribution to health problems. Without such a systematic, structured and quantitative methodology, the identification of causes and provision of solutions would rely on "expert opinion" alone. Although professional opinion is invaluable, it is helpful to provide supporting evidence of cost-benefits to justify design changes. The last point is particularly important for the smaller business where investment in redesign is subject to relatively small budgets being available for such purposes.

LITERATURE FINDINGS

The literature was examined for design criteria as an initial step in developing an ergonomic approach to minimising the occurrence of ULSI. Examples include: "Keep the wrist straight while rotating forearm and hand" (Tichauer, 1976) and: Provide "proper instruction and continued supervision of each worker" (Hymovitch and Lindholm, 1966). Although such recommendations are sound general advice, they do not provide a quantitative basis for criteria of acceptability or practical assistance for equipment redesign.

Clearly, there is a need for the development of criteria which specify the biomechanical limitations of the upper limbs in relation to posture, force and repetition rates. Task elements containing actions exceeding such criteria should be examined in more detail. Examination of the actions in which combinations of force, posture and repetition occurred could eventually provide an index from which to establish priorities for specifying those elements which put the worker most at risk.

METHODOLOGY
Developing Working Criteria

The ULSI literature had little to offer by way of quantitative guidelines so other literature sources were examined for their suitability. The 5th percentile maximum voluntary movement cited by Harris and Harris (1968) was chosen to set a range of movements which would be tolerated by a high percentage of the working population. A further reduction to 75% of the 5th percentile value was chosen so that those with 5th percentile limits in their movement would not be disadvantaged. Also these values were selected as a compromise between the requirement for some realistic movement and literature recommendations which said that there should be no movement. Criteria for isometric muscular effort (Rohmert, 1960) and repetitive muscular effort (Moelbech, 1963) were obtained in a similar way.

Using these, it allows the ergonomist to assess the loadings on the hand and arm against objective values. It also provides a method of quantifying recommendations, for example, "reduce this angle by twenty degrees" or "break the static load every 2 minutes". This approach makes the results of any field study immediately useful to the client because priorities for change can be readily identified as well as the types of change needed.

The Industrial Context

For these criteria to be of practical utility, there had to be a method of collecting data from jobs which had to be usable in a range of industries, locations and within the budgetary constraints of a variety of companies. Four features are required:

(i) it must be inexpensive for the client;
(ii) it must be applicable within the workplace;
(iii) it must provide a structured approach to identify those features which contribute to the problem;
(iv) it must assist in determining priorities for action by the client.

The initial step was to identify techniques which would provide postural, force and repetition data. There was no readily available system to measure forces. Trials were carried out with a experimental system of mercury-filled strain gauges to provide postural data.

Practical rather than technical factors limited the use of the technique. These were portability, the need for an on-site mains power supply, the risk of contamination to product, preparation time and the space required on-site.

It was concluded that a methodology would need to be developed which did not depend upon instrumentation with these shortcomings.

Development of the Methodology

It was decided that the simplest and most practical way of obtaining data was to record the task on video and derive as many values as possible from the playback ("synthetic real time analysis"). Pilot studies indicated that it would be possible to collect and interpret postural intervals as fine as 5 degrees. Direct observation of the subject tends to be faster and easier because the observer has the benefit of being able to view in three dimensions and has mobility to alter the view. In order to ensure that data can be checked, it is also advisable to video record. However, in a number of situations there is insufficient time on-site to do both, so video was adopted as the recording method. The collection of angular data is based on sampling the extremes of the postures of wrist, elbow and shoulder at each of these points. Sustained postures are also noted and quantified for comparison with isometric criteria. This level of accuracy copes with individual variations in style and also is capable of distinguishing between different jobs.

Quantifying Force

Knowledge about which aspects of the force(s) applied by the upper limbs contributes to ULSI is limited. The consensus of opinion is that maintenance of unvarying force over time results in high loads being imposed on the musculoskeletal system. This is judged to be a particular problem where such forces are found in conjunction with excessive joint angles.

The Institute's experience in studies to-date shows that there is little to be gained from measuring forces in most preliminary field surveys. Apart from the fact that there are technical difficulties in getting such data, analysis of video measurement can indicate if the duration of the force is likely to be a potentially critical factor. Until the importance of force as a contributory factor has been determined, objective measurement of force is not a primary study requirement. If this information is needed, then it is possible to obtain it from simulation trials away from the workplace.

Quantifying Rates of Work

Video measurement permits timing of the activity away from the workplace. Cycle times, task element times, durations of force applied and rest periods in the cycle were measured quickly and easily. These values were used in conjunction with the angle, force and discomfort data to give an indication of the relative task loadings arising from the job, equipment or methods.

The duration of static loading in the task cycle (for example, in using a tool) was of particular interest. The data were expressed as percentages of cycle length for isometric loading, and in conjunction with force estimates from other studies in the literature to assess stress. Examining the sequence of task elements indicated whether a static force was being applied while the wrist was in motion and the extent of that motion. Presentation of this data with time values showed management, in a simple form, which sequence of events may be contributing to ULSI and so provided a systematic means of identifying causal factors which would require alteration.

Quantifying Discomfort

An assessment of postural comfort was considered to be a useful complement to the other measures in order to examine the impact of whole body posture on upper limb strain, in particular the shoulder. Subjective assessment of whole body and regional discomfort and their progression with time was required. A variant of the postural comfort diagram (Corlett and Bishop, 1976) with additional regions for the wrist and hand was selected for ease of application. This was a useful comparative tool because the results were available in a graphical form. It was possible to identify the potential for biomechanical problems arising from equipment and task design that needed to be resolved at the same time as the ULSI problems, if the overall level of stress on the hand and arm was to be reduced.

INDUSTRIAL CASE STUDIES

Two examples of the application of the methodology to different industrial situations are outlined below.

Site 1

There had been a number of ULSI cases diagnosed on this site. The safety manager wished to identify possible means of reducing the incidence. However, a major constraint on this study was that the client company was able to fund only a limited investigation. The study was conducted by two persons, in two days on-site, examining eight tasks. The methods used were the whole body and local discomfort questionnaires, workspace measurement, anthropometric measures, video recording and direct measurement of joint angles using simple goniometers. These were compared with criteria developed as described earlier. Tables of the results from 46 questionnaires and 21 task analyses were presented.

The report was used as a basis for discussion with the client. The presentation of data, such as the percentage of task postures exceeding the criteria and illustrations of discomfort zones, assisted management in rapidly comparing one task feature with another. On this basis, it was possible to identify priorities for change. These changes were then examined in relation to the practicality for redesign or implementation of alternative solutions. For example, because of the very small number of jobs in the plant containing features not likely to cause ULSI, it was decided that job rotation would only increase the number of people at risk until equipment and job redesign had taken place. However, before progress could be made the company was sold and several hundred jobs were lost from that plant. As a consequence, the redesign solutions were not pursued.

Site 2

A new assembly line for motor vehicle engines was being designed. The method was applied to simulations of four workstations which the design team suspected would have potential problems in relation to predicted cycle times. Four simulated tasks were studied in 43 different combinations of worker and layout in a two-day study. Video was used as the source of all data and the results were presented a week after the simulations. The results showed that there were some task elements in which postural and repetition criteria and the predicted cycle times were exceeded.

Improved presentation of material and workstation design were identified as ways to reduce the potential stress of the elements of the tasks likely to create health problems. A further benefit of such improvements would be the possibility of reducing task element times to bring the overall cycle within predicted values. Management recognised that the use of an objective ergonomic methodology provided a cost-effective way of evaluating workstation design at an early stage in the design process to identify productivity, health and safety implications of design decisions.

CONCLUSIONS

The success of industrial ergonomics depends on three major factors:

    (i) the availability of evaluation and design criteria;

(ii) the provision of objective information for management decisions;
(iii) being involved at the right time in the design process.

Until the working criteria were developed, it was difficult to identify potential musculoskeletal problems systematically. Although the criteria have not been validated by research, the approach provides a methodology which complements expert opinion. In practice, the structured evaluation and analysis showed quantifiable differences between "high and low risk" jobs. This was sufficient for management to be confident that the effort required to meet the criteria would be justified by reductions in the risk levels and improvements in productivity.

The provision of quantitative results provided a means to assess the priorities for design. The implications of a design change could be presented to management in terms of specific effect on a task element. It was also much easier to identify the contribution which an element made to the musculoskeletal problems. Alterations to product mix and production method could be examined in detail, and manipulated to assess the implications for productivity as well as health and safety.

Costs of production and ability to respond to fluctuating demands are major considerations in day-to-day management decision making. Managers' priorities are to acquire information at the right time to minimise costs and achieve productivity targets. The need to achieve rapid results from a study precludes the use of sophisticated but time-consuming techniques. The time constraint may also limit the choice of technical options for redesign available to management. However, through a structured approach and the use of objective criteria, professional ergonomic opinion and expertise can assist greatly in management decision making. In providing this assistance, there is also a need to ensure that ergonomic data are available in a form which maximises the design team's use of local management expertise as this can reduce the cost and time involved in creating improvements to task or cquipment designs.

The approach adopted by the Institute provides a practical means of minimising the effects of task and workplace design on health, particularly ULSI, until research leading to definitive criteria has been carried out.

REFERENCES

Corlett, E.N. & Bishop, R.B., 1976, A Technique for Assessing Postural Discomfort. Ergonomics; 19: 175-182.

Harris, M.L. & Harris C.W., 1968, A factor analytic study of flexibility. Paper presented to the National Convention of the American Association of Health Physical Education and Recreation, Research Section. St. Louis, Missouri.

Hymovitch, L. & Lindholm, M., 1966, Hand, Wrist and Forearm Injuries: The Result of Repetitive Motions. Journal of Occupational Medicine; 8: 573-577.

Moelbech, S., 1963, "Average Percentage Force at Repeated Maximal Isometric Muscle Contractions at Different Frequencies". Communications from the Testing and Observations Institute of the Danish National Association for Infantile Paralysis; 16: 1963.

Rohmert, W., 1960, "Ermittlung von Erholungspausen fur Statische Arbeit des Menschen". Internationale Zeitschrift fur Angewandte Physiologie; 18: 123.

Tichauer, E.R., 1976, "Biomechanics Sustains Occupational Safety and Health". Industrial Engineering; 8: 45-56.

PATIENT LIFTING: AN ERGONOMIC APPROACH

K.J. Poll

Veiligheidsinstituut
Amsterdam

INTRODUCTION

In most hospitals and nursing-houses we see an increase of the fysical, and mental, workload. Less nurses and a shorter stay of patients mean more heavy work. The sicknessrate, rising in some places, is for a great percentage caused by complaints about neck and shoulder. As in England in Holland this means a loss in days and money (Stubbs e.a. 1984)
Results of different studies on working conditions in nursing show that the lifting of "patients" is one of the greatest risks for the safety and health in nursing. People are heavy and in many situations difficult to grasp. The fysical workload can be minimised by good workplace design and the right lifting-method.
In the poster two different methods are compared and the effect of workplace design improvement is demonstrated. The task that is chosen for this poster is the lifting of a lying patient from the bed on to brancard.

METHOD

For the task two volunteers (185, 189 cm) were asked to lift the patient six times from the bed on to the brancard. They had enough rest and some training. They lifted the patient from one side of the bed in two different ways.
Method 1: arms around the patient.
Method 2: both arms under the back of the patient.

The standard hospitalbed was placed in his highest position (80 cm). Before lifting the patient was moved to the side of the bed. Videorecords were made from the right side of the lifting volunteers. From these records distances were measured.

With the NIOSH-guidelines (NIOSH, 1981) Action Limit and Maximum Permisseble Limit were calculated. For the horizontal distance the centre of gravity was taken. The vertical position was corrected for the facts that the patient was lifted on the arms and not by hand.

For both methods the starting position, the moment the patient left the bed, was taken as moment for the judgement. Experiments showed that both volunteers lifted the same amount of weight (half of the patient) for both methods.

The same lifting task was executed on a experimental bed. This bed had the possibility to place the patient 100 cm from the floor. With the NIOSH-guidelines these situations were also calculated. The volunteers chosed themselves the right height.

RESULTS

The results of the calculated NIOSH-guidelines are summarised in table 1.

Table 1. guidelines for the safe (AL) and maximum permisseble (MPL) patientweight (in kg), for different lifting methods and bedheights.

Lifting method	80 cm AL	MPL	100 cm AL	MPL
1	24	70	28	86
2	18	54	31	94

CONCLUSION AND DISCUSSION

The results show that the height of the bed in relation with the lifting methods determine the risk of patient lifting. The higher position of the bed means for method 2 that the horizontal distances between patient and lifting person is shorter. This is caused by more legroom under the bed and less bending of the back.

Especially at 80 cm, standard bed, there is a difference between the two methods. This difference disappears at 100 cm height.

These results are based on the lifting by two volunteers. More general information can be achieved by an experiment with more persons and more different heights.

For the present the conclusion is that for most nursers and nurses the hospitalbed are to low and that an instruction for lifting methods depends on the lenght of the person or the height of the bed.

LITERATURE

NIOSH, Work Practices Guide for Manual Material Handling. National Instiute for Occupational Health and Safety, 1981.

Stubbs, D.A. and P.W. Buckle, Epidemiology of Back Pain in the Nursing Profession. Nursing 2, 32, 935-938, 1984.

MUSCULOSKELETAL PROBLEMS IN SUPERMARKET WORKERS

G. Anthony Ryan

Occupational Health and Safety Unit
Department of Social and Preventive Medicine
Monash Medical School
Alfred Hospital
Prahran, Victoria, Australia

ABSTRACT

This paper reports a prevalence study of musculo-skeletal symptoms in supermarket workers in Melbourne, Australia, carried out with the Shop, Distributive and Allied Employees Union during 1986. Supermarkets were stratified by number of employees, and a sample of establishments within each stratum visited. Each employee was given a questionnaire which covered personal details, frequency of body posture, movements, equipment use, symptoms, if any, and questions relating to job demand, and job satisfaction. As far as possible, the format of the questions used followed that of a similar study in the U.K. Results of a preliminary analysis of the data, and a comparison with the U.K. study will be presented.

POSTURAL FACTORS, WORK ORGANISATION AND MUSCULOSKELETAL SYMPTOMS

G. ANTHONY RYAN
BRIDGET HAGE
MARGO BAMPTON

Occupational Health and Safety Unit
Department of Social & Preventive Medicine
Monash Medical School
Alfred Hospital
Prahran, Victoria, Australia

In 1983 and 1984 143 data process operators (DPOs) in four data entry sections in Commonwealth Government departments in Melbourne were surveyed using a questionnaire which covered personal details, training, perceptions of job demand, symptoms, if any, and the Work Environment Scale of Insel and Moos[1]. Each DPO was interviewed and had a brief physical examination of neck, shoulder and arms, as well as an ergonomic assessment including measurements of limb angles and distances.

Symptoms were graded according to a six point scale from 0 to 5, according to frequency, with the lower arm, and the shoulder and neck, being given separate scores. These scores were combined, for a possible range of 0 to 10. Forty-one DPOs with scores of 8 or more were classed as the "high" group, and 28 DPOs with scores of two or less were classed as the "low" group, for upper limb symptoms (ULS). This ULS grouping was then used as a dichotomous dependent variable in the subsequent analysis.

Our aim was to examine the effect, singly and together, of posture, perceived job demand, and work social environment on the probability of developing ULS.

The three variables with the largest odds ratio for ULS were selected for each of the three dimensions, posture, Job Demand and Work Environment.(Table 1) These odds ratios were all statistically significant at the 5 percent level, and they were all quite substantial, ranging from 3.2 to 7.7. Within each dimension logit modelling was carried out with the SPSS^X package using the log linear procedure. Within the Job Demand dimension, job stress was dropped from the model, and a joint variable

Table 1. Risks of Upper Limb Symptoms.

Posture	odds ratio	Job Demand	odds ratio	Work Environment	odds ratio
L elbow angle	3.9	Boredom	7.7	Peer cohesion	6.7
Eye-copy distance	3.2	Pushing self	3.9	Staff support	1/4.1
L Shoulder flexion	3.2	Job stress	3.7	Autonomy	3.9

Final Model

	Relative Risk		Relative Risk		Relative Risk
L elbow angle	0	Job Demand		Peer Cohesion	
		High	20		
		Medium	4	- Low	5
		Low	1	- High	1

constructed by combining boredom and pushing self into three categories: high (high on both), medium, (high on one), low (low on both). For Posture, left elbow angle remained as the only variable, and in Work Environment, peer cohesion was selected, all other variables dropping out. Finally, logit modelling was carried out on three remaining variables, which were assumed to be independent. Posture dropped out of the model, as its effect was insignificant. There was a joint effect between Job Demand and Work Environment, the relative risks of the three levels of Job Demand and two levels of Work Environment being shown in Table 1. The effects of these two variables are independent and multiplicative, with a relative risk of 90 being estimated for cases low on Work Environment, and high on Job Demand.

These results suggest that while postural variables have an effect on musculo-skeletal symptoms of the upper limb, these effects are over shadowed by the effects of job demand, and the social climate of the work place. The implication is that attention should be paid to the management and organisation of work, as well as to the physical and ergonomic aspects, in the prevention and management of musculo-skeletal symptoms.

REFERENCES

Moos, R.H. and Insel, P.M. The Work Environment. Scale. Consulting Psychologists Press Inc. Palo Alto, CA. 1974.

ACKNOWLEDGEMENT

The survey was supported by a Health Service Research Grant from the Commonwealth Department of Health.

MUSCULOSKELETAL DISORDERS AT WORK IN BUILDING
CONSTRUCTIONS : EPICONDYLITIS AND LOW BACK PAINS

B. Salengro and F. Commandre*

Medecin du Travail, Apamentra Btp, 6 rue Dr. Richelmi,
06300 Nice, France
*Rhumatologue, 23 bd Carabacel, 06000 Nice, France

INTRODUCTION

The scope of this work is based on the relationship between working conditions and rheumatism.

The link between the number of cases of degenerative rheumatic disease and one's workload has been proved scientifically. We have selected two examples for study - low back pain and epicondylitis.

Our results come from a close collaboration between works' physicians in the building industry and rheumatologists from Nice. These works are the fruit of the methodology that we will develop in the first section. In the second section we will present the results of a study on backache. In the third section, the study deals with epicondylitis, its economic and legal consequences.

METHODOLOGY

The methods used for this study are taken from the results of systematic screening of every French worker annually by works' physicians, sometimes helped by a consultant rheumatologist.

Every French worker has a medical consultation every year in order to:
- look for infectious diseases;
- verify his aptitude for his job;
- search for any elements which could bring
  modifications or change in his job;
- improve working and living conditions in industry
  (safety, health, toxicology, ergonomy).

This systematic examination annually of all workers has also a very big epidemiologic advantage of which we are only now beginning to see the first results.

We can foresee in the near future with the introduction of computers in the medical world, bigger and better results.

The following studies have been realised on the same principle : the grouping together of the people concerned by this illness, and to compare this with the general population regarding professional characteristics given by administrative reports : age, seniority, job.

These jobs are then studied from a physiological point of view to verify the logical development of this illness : articular overload, heavy workload, vibrations ... and so on.

STUDY ON THE BACKACHE

During an 18 month period, 4065 workers in the building trades and construction industry were examined. Low back pains were observed in 488 people. The 'backache' criteria was a backache with a professional consequence. It is a diagnosis between the man and his work. By profession, the results are:
- administrators   3.5%   - unskilled workmen   10.0%
- apprentices   4.7%   - professional workmen   14.8%
- staff/foremen   8.4%   - engine drivers   23.1%

A more precise analysis is possible, the results being:
- drivers of heavy   - mechanics   24.3%
  machinery   30.6%
- bricklayers   21.0%   - roofing felt layers   30.7%
- plumbers/heating
  workers   22.0%

These two statements show incontestable differences of frequency, connected with the type of work.

A more precise analysis comes with age:

Fifty per cent of low back pain sufferers are aged between 40 and 50 years for drivers of heavy machinery and mechanics.

After between 20 and 30 years of working life, nearly 50% of mechanics and nearly 40% of heavy machinery drivers suffer low back pain.

The same is found for the 137 house builders with low back pain. The peak on the graph is at 48% for those aged between 25 and 30 years old.

STUDY ON EPICONDYLITIS

Writer's cramp (Runge 1873), tennis elbow (Morris 1882), the famous name and its success, overuse (Remark 1894), fencing masters accident (Couderc 1896), tennis-Schmerz (Bahr 1900), tennis arm (Clado 1902) and epicondylalgia or epicondylitis (rheumatologists and sports physicians).

These different names are found in the literature in studies of the frequently occurring disease of the elbow : epicondylitis. The connection between an occupation (work or sport) and this disease is very often observed by the authors. The nine works' physicians completed a questionnaire each time they encountered a case of epicondylitis and this information was analysed by computer based on 13,458 examinations.

If we compare each column of the histogram of results, we see that from the number of workers examined, 49% were manual workers. Of the sufferers of epicondylitis, 83% were building site workers. The distribution difference between the two populations can be tested by the X^2 pearson confirming it by 1%. We may complete this study by checking the distribution of epicondylitis amongst professional workmen (see illustration).

We also notice a large difference according to occupations, particularly 33.7% of epicondylitis amongst brick-layers, who only represent 14.59% of the workers in the building industry. It is even more evident with the front house's builders (personnel who apply cement rendering by trowel projection) where 10.3% of epicondylitis sufferers are found, while they only represent 0.11% of the building workers. Fifty-seven per cent of the front house builders during this period were found to be suffering from epicondylitis.

RETROSPECTIVE STUDY

After studying 35 patients known to be suffering from epicondylitis during a period of four years from 1977 to 1981, the following information was extracted:

Professional building workers take first place, as they represent 52% of all visits, (a reminder that they represent 15% of our patients). Of these 52% the building personnel who apply cement rendering to houses (front house builder) part-time or full-time, 29% were found to suffer from epicondylitis.

Another point of view, from medical reports, concerns two different types of jobs, front house builders (50) (or cement renderers) and steel workers (173) the percentages were 32% and 1.1%.

PHYSIOLOGICAL STUDY

This consists of analysing the professional movements of the front house builders. The results show:
 - the frequency of supination and of extension of the

forearm,
- the importance of heavy workload.
* every minute 23kg of material are handled and thrown,
* during one day we evaluate the total weight to be about six tons.

The legal aspect: because of the demonstration of a professional link, it was asked that epicondylitis be recognised as a professional illness, in order to give adequate pensions to these workers, and to provoke a change in the working habit.

Distribution of populations according to the type of job
dark : epicondylitis sufferers white : building worker in general.

Pl : Plasterer
Pe : Painter
Ma : Brick Layer
Fa : Front House Builder
Co : Moulder

CONCLUSION
These two examples show that epidemiologic studies are useful because to be obliged to repair is the best way to be obliged to prevent. We hope that with the introduction of a more intensive use of medical software by the works'

physicians more intensive and deeper studies will be achieved.

AUTHOR INDEX

Adams, P.K. 183
Akinmayowa, N.K. 189, 194
Akintunji, I. 194
Andersen, V 68, 82
Andersson, R. 146

Bammer, G 118, 200
Bampton, M. 251
Barch Holst,U. . 110
Baxter, C.E. 165
Biering-Sorensen, F. 68, 82
Bjurvald, M. 146
Blader,S. . 110
Blignault, I. 118
Boss,A.H. 68, 82
Broersen,J. 17
Brown, D. 165
Browne, K. 43
Buchalter, D. . 171
Buckle,P.W. 102, 124
Byfield, D. 201

Carbone,A, 25
Clark, A.G. 43
Colombini,D. 89
Commandre,F. 254
Cristofolini,A. 89

Danielsson, S. 110
de Vries,M. 17
Dorsky, S. . 171
Dul,J. 227

Eklund, J.A.E. 50, 56, 62
Ellis, N. 139

Ferhm, E. . 110
Fine, L.J. 31, 74, 108
Foreman, T.K. 165

Gracovetsky,S 25
Graves, R.J. 183, 239
Grieco, A. 89

Hage, B. 251
Hasan, J, 23
Hildebrandt, V. 9

Josefsen,K. 68, 82

Kahanovitz, N. 171, 213, 234
Kalpamaa,M. . 110
Kasdan,M.L. 133
Kemmlert, K. . 146
Keyserling,W.M. 31, 74, 108
Kilbom, A. . 146
Kompier,M. 17
Kumar, S, 37

Leijon, M. 110
Leino,P. 23
Liddicoat, K. 139
Lindh,M. 110
Lortie, M. 159
Lowerson,A. 177

Mabey, M.H. 183, 239
Madeley, R 43
Markhede,G 110
Meijman,T. 17
Meyer, R.H. 112
Mikaelsson, B. 110
Moritz,U. 234
Mulders,H. 17
Mulvihill,M. 213

Nakata,M. 221
Nishiyama, K 221
Nijboer,I 227
Nilsson, B. . 146
Nordin, M. 171, 213, 234

Occhipinti,E. 89
Odenrick, P. 50, 56, 62
Ortengren, R. 56

Parnianpour,M. 213, 234
Pethick, A.J. 183, 239
Poll, K.J. 247
Porter,R.W. 75
Punnett, L. 31, 74, 108

Ridd, J.E. 43
Ryan, A. 250, 251

Salengro,B 254
St-Vincent, M. . 159
Stubbs, D.A. 102

Tellier, C. 159
Thompson, D. 177
Troup,J.D.G. . 165
Turner, J.P. 124

van der Grinten, M. 96
van Noord,F. 17
Vincent, M. 102
Viola, K. 213

Waersted, M. 153
Watanabe,S. 221
Westgaard, R.H. 153

Yabut,S. 213

Zalewski,M. 177
Zettergren, S. 50, 56, 62

SUBJECT INDEX

accidents, 68
activity analysis, 43

back disorders, 74
back injury, 68, 82
back load, 96
back pain, 75, 189
biomechanical stress, 31
bricklayers, 189
bus drivers, 17

cargo handlers, 194
Carpal Tunnel Syndrome 124, 133
case-referent study, 74 ,108
clerical workers, 112
computer data acquisition, 43
construction industry, 254
crane cabin design, 62
crane drivers, 62

data process operators, 251
demographic trends, 82
diagnosis of low back pain, 201
disc height, 25
dynamic anthropometry, 56
dynamic strength measures, 37

electrical stimulation, 213
engineering industry, 23
epicondylitis, 254
epidemiology, 9 ,82
ergonomics 189, 194
ergonomic redesign, 183

female trunk strength, 234
food processing industry, 183
freight container tractor
   drivers, 221
furniture industry, 227

goniometers, 56

Hettinger Test, 177
history of low back pain, 165
hospital equipment, 247
hospital workers, 159

individual characteristics, 75
intervention study, 146
isokinetic strength, 37, 234
isometric strength, 37, 234

job design, 37

keyboard operators, 200

locomotion, 25
low back pain, 165, 221, 254
lumbar brace, 171
lumbar corset, 171

manual working capacity, 165
metal industry, 23
methodological approaches 9
muscle strength, 213

neck disorders, 110

nurses, 247

occupational diseases, 68
occupational neurosis, 112
oil industry, 153
operators, 110

patient lifting, 247
pelvis and spine biomechanics, 25
physical examination, 201
physical work environment, 17
postural analysis, 62
postural stress, 89
posture analysis, 31, 43
predictors, 165
prevention, 139, 146, 183
psychophysical ratings, 102
Pyridoxine, 133

quarrymen, 89

reach requirements, 37
Repetition Strain Injury, 112, 118, 139, 153, 200
repetitive strain, 189
review, 9, 118, 124
risk factors for RSI, 118
risk factors for back pain, 75
role of physical workload, 23

screening, 177
seated work, 50
sewing machine, 110
shoulder disorders, 108, 110
shoulder elevation, 108
shovel design, 96
spinal compression, 31
spinal diseases, 89
spinal immobilization, 171
spinal shrinkage, 102
standing aids, 227
supermarket workers, 250

task analysis, 50, 239
tenosynovitis, 177
training in lifting techniques, 159
treatment, 133
treatment for RSI, 118
trunk posture, 74

upper limb strain, 183, 239
upper limb symptoms, 251
use of lifting techniques, 159

vibration, 221
Vitamin B6, 133

work organization 153, 251
work strain, 17